CONSIDER THIS —

recovering harmony and balance naturally

CONSIDER THIS —
recovering harmony and balance naturally

Ayn W. Cates, PhD

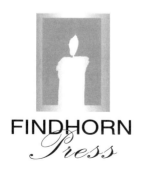

FINDHORN
Press

British Library Cataloguing-in-Publication Data.
A catalogue record for this book is available
from the British Library.

Set in Palatino by Findhorn Press
Illustrations © Gwen Cates 1995
Cover illustration© Gwen Cates 1995
Author photograph by Suzanna Crampton
Cover design by Posthouse Printing
Printed and bound by Cromwell Press Ltd,
Melksham, England

Published by
Findhorn Press
The Park, Findhorn,
Forres IV36 0TZ, Scotland
01309-690582 / fax 690036
e-mail thierry@findhorn.org

Let him

who does not understand

be silent

or learn.

— *John Dee*

Acknowledgements

I would like to thank Dottie Hook for the inspiration and love behind this book. She is a walking light for so many on this earth. I would also like to thank Colin Ryder-Richardson for supporting me and steering me in the right direction. Thanks must be extended to Steve Hellaby who has offered a lot of assistance and support. Thanks also to Sue Shattock and the beautiful afternoon when the title of the book was born. Thanks must also be extended to Patsy Westworth for organising me, to Suzanna Crompton for the wonderful photograph and to Vicky Kerr for supporting me emotionally. Thanks also to Gwen Cates for the imaginative illustration and Bill Cates for assistance on the homeopathy chapter. Finally, I would like to thank Andrew St George for his contribution and love.

Introduction

Consider this —
recovering harmony and balance naturally

> *If you stick to logic you cannot go very far. What is logic other than the conventional way of thinking at a particular time and place?*
> —*Daskalos*

This book has been written for both practitioner and patient, mindful that we have no absolute nor certain knowledge – we are always continuing to learn. Yesterday's medical heresy can be today's truth. We now understand that we are all unique individuals and that what works for one person may not work for another.

When we are sick, or when we are looking after those who are critically ill, it is often difficult to amass reliable information about alternative or complementary therapies. This workbook is designed to do that for you. It will help guide you to the therapy or therapies of most interest to you and provide contact information and useful references for those who wish to study in greater depth. Many of these therapies can be used safely and effectively at home. However, it is always wise to contact an experienced health practitioner or to locate a local healing group where you can share your experience.

The way to begin is with positive thinking. Your thought patterns create your reality. Discipline your thoughts through meditation, auto-suggestion and balanced nutrition and it is likely that you will discover a new happier and healthier self. I am offering you insight into your current state of health – not one of sickness, but one of well-being. The work is up to you. I am inviting you to take responsibility for your own reality and state of being.

Begin now with the realisation that the body is always trying to maintain itself in a condition of good health.

If it is not in good health then ask yourself why and listen to the small voice inside that answers. What obstacles have we set in the way of good health? Thoughtless dietary habits, an unhealthy environment, a mind–body conflict? We begin to heal the body when we remove the mental and physical impediments to health. Good health begins with taking full responsibility for our body–mind–spirit. When we begin to direct the mind (or our mental, emotional and spiritual aspects), we invite beneficial effects at the physical level.

The idea that we live in a world that is alive is fundamental to life in the twentieth century. Self-healing begins when we become aware of the world and learn to live in harmony with it. What is happening within us (both our levels of harmony and disease) is also reflected in our relationships. We can also see this mirrored in world affairs. What is happening to us is also happening in the world of spirit. We live in a holographic universe.

The main focus of this workbook is to awaken the inner tuition and the power of love within each of us since these build the foundations for any type of healing.

We live in a world that day by day grows increasingly challenging and interesting. On one hand, we have to deal with more and more stress – our physical bodies are stressed by our polluted environment and we are mentally and emotionally stressed by a bombardment of information and competitive human interaction. On the other hand, we have rediscovered some of the wisdom of the ancients and have also made new discoveries that benefit our health and well-being.

Many people today are looking for survival techniques, others simply want to enhance their lives. In this workbook I hope to help you with both. The intention is to assist you in developing and discovering the power of self-healing, as well as providing you with useful information on alternative healing. I also hope that as you become familiar with each of the twelve sections of this book, your life will become more harmonious and fulfilled. I want to share this information with you so that you can take what you have learned and assist in the awakening of this beautiful planet and in the healing of yourself and others.

The basic skills

The basic skills you will learn — and be able to pass on — include an introduction to twelve alternative therapies with practical skills and applications from each: aromatherapy & massage, colour therapy, crystal healing, flower essences, homoeopathy & tissue salts, nutritional medicine, energy therapies, reflexology, sound therapy, spiritual healing, visualisation & meditation techniques and yoga.

One of the best ways to develop your awareness is writing. I ask that you keep a daily journal while going through this workbook. Five natural writing exercises are supplied for you to experiment with. I encourage you to explore the intuitive feminine right-hand side of the brain that has been neglected for so long. The twelve sections are divided by astrological symbols. You may like to begin with your sun or moon sign, or the image that most appeals to you. Explore the book at your own pace and in the order that interests you. For instance, if flower essences interest you, turn straight to that section. Let your higher self or intuition guide you.

It is time to tap into your innate wisdom – the force that will transform you and thus transform the world. This requires listening to the noises around you: an aeroplane, the wind in the trees, a bird in full song. Listen to the song that lies beyond that. You are a song within the great orchestra of the universe. The trick is in tapping into that melody. It requires both patience and dedication.

Table of Contents

Foreword

Ayn Cates is a member of our Charity "New Approaches to Cancer". She was asked if she would write a workbook for students who wished to discover their own healing powers through Alternative or Complementary Medicine. This book is the result and we are pleased to recommend it to you the reader. Thank you, Ayn.

Out of a possible hundred or so subjects, Ayn was invited to write on twelve of her choice. This book is her free expression and personal views. As you read the book you will discover much about the work we do and will surely have been inspired by Ayn.

You may not wholly understand all that is written, but as a student you will expect that, there is much to absorb. Just know that every person treads their own path of self discovery. If you feel stimulated to go further then use this book as a blueprint for your own growth.

"BASIC AWARENESS CORRESPONDENCE COURSE."
Our charity will run a course, the cost of which will be small as all the research etc. will be in your hands. Every month you will send us an essay and at the end of a year your knowledge will have grown. Providing this cultivation is competent then we will send you a Certificate.

If this idea sews a seed in your mind and you want to germinate it, then tell us about yourself and your ambitions. Providing what you tell us is satisfactory, we will invite you to choose your twelve subjects.

Please write to me at the address below.

Colin Ryder Richardson

NEW APPROACHES TO CANCER
Through Positive Self Help

Colin Ryder Richardson
5 Larksfield
Egham
Surrey
TW20 0RB
Tel: (01784) 433610
Registered Charity No. 285530

Introduction to workbook for those with an immune system imbalance

Our natures are the physicians of our diseases.
– Hippocrates

In this workbook I hope to provide some information about safe and natural alternatives to orthodox medicine. Many non-toxic methods are often considered unscientific. What difference does that make? Generally speaking, you have everything you need within yourself to make you whole and well. The trick is in becoming aware of it.

There are many cancer treatments that have been tried and tested over the years. One example is the Hoxsey treatment, a combinations of herbs (poke root, burdock root, barberry or *Berberis* root, buckthorn bark, stillingia root – also known as queen's yaw or silver root – and prickly ash bark) which has been used as an unconventional cancer treatment for nearly 100 years. Hoxey's chain of American clinics were shut down by US medical authorities but his treatment still survives at the Tijuana, Mexico, Bio-Medical Center. There are many other treatments available. However, at present there is no single method that has been proven to cure cancer every time, but many people have been helped by one method or another.

Hippocrates (5th century B.C.) said, 'Let your food be your medicine and your medicine your food'. We are just beginning to realise the force and wisdom behind these words. Medical scientists are only discovering the many powerful healing qualities of food . . . .

Vitamin A strengthens the immune system and protects the thymus gland (important for immunity). Fish liver oil is one of the richest sources of vitamin A, but should not be taken in excess. It is also found in celery leaves, aubergines, sweet corn, dandelions, parsley, watercress, egg yolks, pumpkin, squash, carrots, tomatoes, sprouted seeds, cream and butter. *Beta-carotene* is a natural chemical found in many brightly coloured fruits and vegetables such as carrots, mangoes, papayas and yams, as well as, green leafy vegetables such as beet greens, spinach and broccoli. Recent research has shown that beta-carotene reduces the risk of cancer. It supports the immune system directly and also provides a source from which the body can make as much vitamin A as it needs. Beta-carotene is quite harmless and is probably the best way of providing vitamin A without risk.

The *B vitamins* are known for their ability to maintain health since they support the body's nervous system and immune function. They are produced naturally by the body; however, they can be destroyed by substances such as alcohol, coffee, drugs, etc. Good natural sources of B vitamins include brewer's yeast, liver and whole grain cereals[1].

Vitamin C is the vitamin which has produced the most impressive results in both reducing the risk of cancer and treating cancer. It aids tissue growth and repair, assists the functioning of the adrenal glands and gives us healthy gums. It can be found in lemons, oranges, grapefruit, red and green peppers, mustard greens, broccoli, kale, paprika, parsley, blackcurrants, cauliflower, cabbage and chives.

Bioflavonoids (vitamin P) are colourful substances often found alongside vitamin C. They include citrin, hesperidin and rutin. Bioflavonoids are found in the white pulp of citrus fruits, grapes, buckwheat, cherries, blackberries and rose hips. Scientists have found that they remove toxic copper from the body and protect vitamin C levels.

Vitamin D is manufactured in the body by exposure to sunlight. Scientists have found that vitamin D, in combination with the mineral calcium, plays an important role in preventing several different types of cancer, particularly cancer of the colon[2]. However, vitamin D can be toxic in more than 50,000 units a day. So again, it's back to diet. Dietary sources include fish liver oil, eggs[3], animal fats, cow's milk, sprouted seeds/grains/legumes, oysters and fish. Some scientists now believe that twenty minutes of sunlight every day is necessary to supply the body with sufficient *vitamin D*. A study at John Hopkins University by Cedric and Frank Garland concluded that brief daily exposure to sunlight helped to prevent cancer[4]. Interestingly enough, they also found that using sun lotions or creams may actually promote the occurrence of cancer. It is not healthy to live indoors, or to sunbathe covered in oils on the beach. Again, we find that a balanced approach is needed.

Vitamin E is found abundantly in wheat germ, cottonseed and palm oils, as well as in other grains, nuts, seeds and legumes (for example, in brown rice, cornmeal, oatmeal and dry beans) and also in lettuce, sweet potatoes, eggs, milk and liver. Scientists have shown that a deficiency can produce sterility in rats. Vitamin E has been shown to reduce the toxicity of chemotherapy.

Vitamin K is essential for both blood clot formation and liver function. The vitamin is generally produced in the body by bacteria in the intestines. Natural sources are alfalfa, green leafy vegetables, kelp, milk, egg yolks, molasses, safflower and other polyunsaturated fats (e.g. olive oil) and yoghurt.

The question of whether or not you can get all of your vitamins and minerals from your diet alone should be discussed with your health practitioner. Certainly it is the safest way to obtain advice on your particular needs. Meanwhile, please supplement your diet with the foods mentioned. It is thought that due to current mass-market agricultural practices (e.g. applying only nitrogen, phosphorous and potassium on crops) many essential elements and micronutrients are missing from our food supply. Therefore, some people may need vitamin and mineral supplements, especially those whose parents have (had) cancer or who are over fifty.

Various *minerals* are also required by the body. Some are toxic in excess, so it is very important to keep in mind your body's individual needs. *Calcium* is the mineral required by the body in greatest abundance, almost all of which goes to building and maintaining a healthy skeletal system. Calcium is found in milk and dairy products, almonds, sesame seeds, cooked greens (for instance kale), molasses, broccoli and tofu.

Magnesium is a mineral that is said to have a beneficial effect in cases of cancer. It is found in fresh green vegetables, wheat germ, soyabeans, whole grains, seafood, figs, corn, apples and oil-rich seeds, nuts and almonds.

A balanced amount of *selenium* in the body has also been linked to low cancer rates. Selenium is said to enhance the body's normal anti-cancer immunity. It is naturally found in brewer's yeast, cereals, broccoli, celery, brazil nuts, mushrooms, dairy products, fish, shellfish, grains, and organ and muscle meats.

Zinc is essential for health. It is found in brewer's yeast, pumpkin seeds, wheat bran and whole-grain products. Men store large amounts of zinc in their prostate glands. There is some controversy whether or not there is a link between zinc deficiency and cancer of the prostate.

The most ancient method of treating cancer is through the use of herbs. Our knowledge takes us back to the beginnings of human history – to the early Egyptians, Amerindians and the Chinese. The aloe plant is known for its soothing effect on cuts and burns, but it also has an amazing ability to boost the immune system. Astragalus is another non-toxic herb known for its ability to boost the immune system. It also is known to ease or minimise the side-effects of chemotherapy. Please see an experienced health practitioner before taking any of these products.

Ayur-Veda or Ayurvedic medicine is an ancient form of herbal medicine that originated in India several thousand years ago. A Harvard-trained MD, Deepak Chopra, is its most prominent advocate. Ayurvedic medicine emphasises that every person and every person's illness is unique. Diseases arise from an imbalance in the body's immune mechanism. Ayurvedic tradition sees mental and emotional factors as critical in causing such imbalances. Ayurvedic practitioners generally read the pulse in order to diagnose. They use herbal compounds, known as rasayanas, for people with cancer in order to boost the immune system and promote longevity.

Cannabis – or marijuana – has been found useful in fighting nausea and other side-effects of conventional chemotherapy. This is obviously a controversial issue.

Other forms of herbal treatment for cancer include chaparral (a type of tea prepared from a perennial evergreen shrub of the American South-West), Chinese herbs, Essiac (a mixture containing mostly four herbs: burdock, indian rhubarb, sorrel and slippery elm), garlic, ginseng (a Chinese cure-all), green tea, Kampo (the Japanese version of traditional Chinese medicine), Kombucha (a naturally fermented drink made from a fungus that prevents chronic disease), Pau d'Arco (a tea made from the inner bark of a tree found in South American rain forests) and spices, which can have surprising anti-cancer effects, especially turmeric.

There are many natural therapies to support and build up the body's natural immunity. Diet, without a doubt, plays a very important role in this process. Section VII of this workbook deals with nutritional medicine and takes into consideration diets, particularly macrobiotics, as a way to health. However, we still maintain that the needs of each individual vary enormously. We urge you to listen to what it is that your body is trying to tell you. In this workbook you will discover ways to 'tune in' to your self – and by doing so we hope you will bring yourself from a state of disease into a state of harmony and balance. This book is not designed to take the place of medical treatment or advice; it is meant to supplement the information that is already widely available.

---

[1] Some research has shown that yeast or liver should not be taken in excessive quantities by people with cancer since B vitamins in certain cases have stimulated tumour formation.

[2] Reference: Ralph W. Moss, PhD, *Cancer Therapy: the independent consumer's guide to non-toxic treatment and prevention*, New York: Equinox, 1992.

[3] A better source would be free-range eggs.

[4] Ralph W. Moss,op. cit., p. 67.

Some useful books for cancer patients

Ralph W Moss, PhD, *Cancer Therapy: the independent consumer's guide to non-toxic treatment and prevention*, New York: Equinox Press, 1992.

Sir Jason Winters, *The Jason Winters Story*, Las Vegas: Vinton Publishing, 1990.

Barry Lynes, *The Healing of Cancer: the cures – the cover-ups and the solution now!*, Canada: Marcus Books, 1989.

Max Gerson, MD, *A Cancer Therapy: results of fifty cases and the cure of advanced cancer by diet therapy: a summary of 30 years of clinical experimentation*, California: The Gerson Institute, 1990.

Dr Peter Mansfield and Dr Jean Monro, *Chemical Children: how to protect your family from harmful pollutants*, London: Century, 1988.

Norman Cousins, *Head First: the biology of hope and the healing power of the human spirit*, London: Penguin, 1990.

Useful addresses

Cancer Help Centre, Grove House, Cornwallis Grove, Clifton, Bristol BA8 4PG. Tel: 01272-743216.

New Approaches to Cancer, Colin Ryder-Richardson, 5 Larksfield, Egham TW20 0RB.

One of the great free human activities ...

Writing is one of the great, free human activities. There is scope for individuality, and elation, and discovery.
– William Stafford

Writing exercise 1

If you can form letters on a page, know the basic structure of a sentence and can write a short thank you note to a friend, then you have all the skills necessary for this workbook. Please do not worry about grammar or spelling. All you need to develop is an attitude of wonder.

In order to chart your own progress, date each entry and keep your writing together in a manila folder or binder. Use paper and pens that suit you. If you prefer to type, that is fine. By the end of the workbook you should be pleased to discover a thick folder of your own writing. Feel free to immerse yourself in the creative process.

It is best to set a time aside each day for writing, for instance, first thing in the morning, at lunch or just before bed when the house is quiet. In the beginning, limit yourself to ten minutes for each of the five entries below. Select one each day in any order, or write about something else that is currently resting on your heart. The important thing is to write, to communicate, to explore both the logical and intuitive parts of the mind.

1. Write about yourself as a child.
2. Write about a conflict that you experienced today (or an unresolved conflict from the past). How does it make you feel? Think of the ways in which you can bring forgiveness to the situation.

3. Describe a feeling such as fear, love, anger or joy.

4. Describe the wind and how it makes you feel.

5. Write about your best friend. (He or she can be imaginary.)

Writing exercise 2

> *Hope is believing in spite of the evidence
> and working toward changing the
> evidence.*
> *– Anon*

1. Take out a sheet of paper and write down a list of things that you feel keep you from living in a balanced state: 'I am limited because... or I can't be healthy because... (e.g. I am limited because I have got to earn a living and I hate my job' or 'I can't be healthy because no one in my family is'). Write as much on this piece of paper (or papers) as you can think of. Be honest with yourself.

2. Then take the paper and dispose of it however you care to: burn it, chew it up, flush it down the toilet, bury it, throw it in the bin, etc. Be as simple or as elaborate as you like.

3. Take out a new sheet of paper and some coloured pens or crayons (if you have some) and colour in these words:

> *I AM HAPPY. I AM HEALTHY.*
> *I AM WEALTHY. I AM FREE.*

Draw each letter with a different colour. Draw butterflies or rainbows, or any image that comes into your mind, into and around the words. Feel the words becoming alive.

4. Hang your drawing up somewhere (maybe on the refrigerator door) where you will see it often and be reminded of its message.

5. Then, to the tune of 'If You're Happy and You Know It' (or another song that you prefer) sing at least once a day: 'I am happy, I am healthy, I am free! I am happy, I am wealthy, I am free! I am happy, I am healthy, I am happy, I am wealthy, I am happy, I am healthy, I am free!'

Writing exercise 3

> *The New Age ego marches to a different drumbeat than those who cling to the past. Their only authority will be within and not in the outer world of appearance. It will be the spirit and not the form that will be of importance.*
> *– Isabell M. Hickey*

Each one of us is completely responsible for our own experiences. Our thoughts have created our past and our present. What we are thinking now is creating our future. In order to manifest what we want in our lives, we must concentrate on the present moment. We create our diseases; we create our well-being. It's time to let go and forgive ourselves and each other. When we find our balance then we find our power. It is at this point that we begin directing our energies effectively. Our task is to become co-creators. Let's begin now.

Take out some coloured pencils and write out an affirmation in your own words. Here is an example:

> *I believe I have celestial guidance*
> *as I walk my golden path.*
> *I believe in miracles,*
> *angels*
> *and unicorns.*

I believe
my physical, emotional
and spiritual bodies are healthy –
that I am safe and protected,
yet free.

I am open to my spiritual partner,
he is also open
to my loving embrace.
We are able to strengthen each other in physical love
and independence.

I know that correct prosperity
will always flow through me
and to me.
I know I am a part of God/Goddess/All That Is.

Without hesitation
I accept my role in the Divine Plan.

Writing exercise 4

> *When we were little we had no difficulty*
> *sounding the way we felt; thus most little*
> *children speak and write with a real*
> *voice.*
> *– Peter Elbow*

It is likely that some of the exercises were easier for you than others. Was it difficult to write about yourself? Now we would like to introduce a simple way of opening the doorway to your intuitive mind.

None of us lacks ideas, but many of us have trouble getting in touch with them. 'Clustering' is the magic key to natural writing. It helps us bypass the logical mind (the left hemisphere of the brain) and puts us in touch with the right hemisphere where we find day-dreams, images and sensations. Clustering is similar to brainstorming or free association. Through clustering we tap into the part of our brain where all the experiences of our lifetime dwell. It opens the door to wonder and creativity.

A word or short phrase acts as the centrepiece or stimulus for recording all the associations that spring to mind in a very short space of time. Clustering always unfolds from a centre, like the ripples that move outward when a child throws a pebble into a pond.

This process will help to remove the barriers to natural writing that happened when you learned grammar at school. Writing should always be fun. Look at the example before attempting your own.

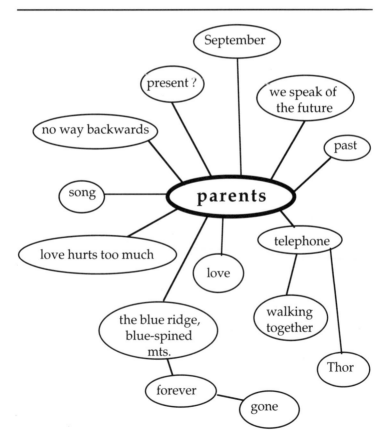

This is an example of clustering revolving around the word 'parents'. The clustering took a maximum of two minutes and the following poem was completed within fifteen minutes. A few words have been changed over the course of time:

September

1
You called me while I was drawing,
reluctantly I followed you
through the new path you had cut.
Five of us spoke a September song
as the fragile autumn leaves
formed a carpet beneath our feet.
For an hour we walked together
looking at the same blue-spined ridge.

2
I did not bother to take a photograph
of Thor's copper chestnut coat
as the sun set behind the pond
and the geese rose in the distance.
He would be there forever, I thought,
as I hurried to meet the train.

When I returned he was dead,
so young and vital and yet he died
from a twisted gut
while my father tried to hold him up
crying, I will never have another horse,
I will never love again.
It hurts too much.

3
Each day after school
my father and I grasped the post-hole digger,
brown bagged the peach brandy

and strode out to tackle the stone infested soil.
It was time to talk,
always mentioning the future
not the present.

Other people live in that house now.
The fruit trees, planted with such care,
have been dismantled, along with our arena
that took us years to build.

4
Now by telephone
we play at togetherness
remembering our home,
pretending we could return
and yet knowing each step we take leads us further away
from that day when we looked
at the blue-spined ridge
and were together.[1]

You are not responsible for any particular order of ideas; no information need come across. You do not even have to show this to anyone, unless you want to. Just let the associations come, and if they don't, then just doodle until they do. When you get a sudden sense of what you want to write about, then simply begin writing. It's easy.

1. Write the word 'BIRTH' in the middle of your page and circle it.

2. Now become playful and allow your mind to make associations.

3. Make connections, but avoid judging or choosing. Simply let go and write.

4. Draw a circle around each word or phrase. Connect with lines the associations that seem related.
5. Keep brainstorming or writing associations for one to

two minutes.

6. Then you will experience a mental shift and realise you have something to write about.

7. If you get stuck, write about anything from the cluster to get you started.

8. Trust yourself.

9. Write for about ten minutes and no more than one and a half to two pages. Include everything you want from your cluster, but try not to stray too far. Use what relates and makes sense.

10. Once you have written your story or poem, bring the piece full circle by ending with your starting idea.

11. Read aloud what you have written.

Seven exercises for clustering

During the next week choose one of these words a day and practice clustering. Include yourself, your world, memories, hopes, dreams, fears, friends, anything that comes to mind. Feel free to choose your own words instead of those supplied. Remember to have fun!

1. RAINBOWS
2. BABY
3. MOON
4. WATER
5. FIRE
6. ANGEL
7. SEA

Writing exercise 5:
Disciplining your Thoughts

> *In most lives insight has been accidental.*
> *We wait for it as primitive man awaited*
> *lightning for a fire. But making mental*
> *connections is our most crucial learning*
> *tool, the essential of human intelligence:*
> *to forge links, to go beyond the given; to*
> *see patterns, relationship, context.*
> *– Marilyn Ferguson*

To learn to meditate effectively you must be able to concentrate well, which requires discipline of thought. Good concentration and clear thinking will benefit many areas of your life, whether you are active in sport, have a mentally demanding job or whatever your daily activities entail. By now you should have established a time and place where you can comfortably meditate on a daily basis.

Writing visualisation

1. Close your eyes and take three deep breaths. Imagine that you are surrounded by bright white light.

2. Now, recall a familiar poem or nursery rhyme. Visualise each word as though it were alive. Repeating the verse in your mind, watch the words and letters escape from your lips and scamper down a corridor like little children.

3. If one tries to wander off, guide it gently back to the corridor. Remember, you are in control.

4. When they reach the end of the corridor (take as long as you wish), ask them to come back to you. Words and

letters have a tendency to scatter unless you concentrate on them. Keep your eyes on all of them. Do not allow your mind to stray until they have all returned to you.

5. Thank them for working with you, then release them.

6. Visualise yourself sitting at your desk. See words and symbols flowing to you. See yourself recording them easily on paper. See yourself smiling. You may even want to imagine a muse or angel standing by your shoulder encouraging you and increasing the powers of your imagination.

7. Wiggle your fingers and toes. Feel yourself back in your body. Please look down before looking up.

I AM

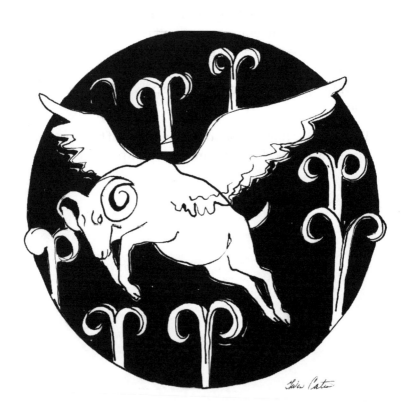

ARIES
"Winged Ram"

I

Aromatherapy and holistic massage

> *The cure of the part should not be attempted*
> *without treatment of the whole, and also no*
> *attempt should be made to cure the body without*
> *the soul, and therefore if the head and body are*
> *to be well you must begin by curing the mind:*
> *that is the first thing... For this is the great error*
> *of our day in the treatment of the human body,*
> *that physicians separate the soul from the body.*
> *– Plato*

Aromatherapy is a healing art that has powerful effects
on mind, body and spirit. The key to aromatherapy lies
in its dual use of essential oils and massage, thus activat-
ing two important senses – smell and touch.

The history of the use of aromatics takes us back
to ancient civilisations, including those of China, Egypt,
India, Arabia and Greece. Egypt was the centre of the sci-
ences, including medicine and perfumery. For example,
fragrant aromatic preparations were found in the tomb of
Tutankhamun[1]. In ancient Egypt, priests were also doctors, and they used numerous combinations of aromatics
for religious ceremonies, as well as for embalming the
dead – the Egyptians believed in reincarnation and they
wanted to keep the body in good condition after death
for its journey to the next life.

In ancient Greece aromatic essences were pre-
scribed to cure illnesses. Hippocrates attempted to halt
the spread of the plague in Athens with aromatic fumi-
gations in the streets.

Aromatic essences fell out of favour with the rise
of Christianity and it was not until the Middle Ages that
they again met with popularity. In the 18th century

essences were often used as a way of fighting epidemics. In the 19th century essences began to be produced synthetically, although in this century there has been a renewed interest in plant extracts and their medicinal qualities.

There are a number of approaches to aromatherapy. The essential oils can be used in baths, burners, inhalers and compresses, or applied to the skin neat (bergamot[2], lavender and ti-tree, only), diluted, or as lotions and creams. Aromatherapeutic foot-baths are often wonderful additions to treatment. A modern aromatherapist will often combine the use of essential oils with reflexology, holistic massage and shiatsu, but do keep in mind that many therapists believe that all three of these therapies should be avoided by cancer patients since they can assist the cancer in spreading via the lymphatic system. Also cancer patients should always dilute the essential oils and avoid using them neat, even lavender. The oils should never be taken internally since they could damage the stomach – they can be absorbed effectively by the skin where they enter the circulatory system, which transports them through the body's internal organs.

The idea behind holism is that, given the chance, the body will heal itself. This means developing a positive mental outlook, enjoying a form of exercise, getting the right amount of sleep, feeling good about yourself, getting proper nutrition and having a spiritual outlet, as well as using aromatic essences and other techniques to protect and enhance the body's immune system.

Essential oils are sometimes referred to as the soul of the plant. On a more mundane level, they are the liquid components of aromatic plants. They come from many sources, e.g. petals (rose), fruit (bergamot), leaves (eucalyptus), wood (sandalwood), seeds (caraway). All aromatic essences have antiseptic and bactericidal properties and some, such as garlic and ti-tree oil, have antiviral and antibiotic properties as well. Unlike chemical anti-septics, essential oils do not harm tissue and yet act as aggressors towards germs. Essential oils stimulate and reinforce the body's innate healing mechanisms. Essences of chamomile and thyme, for example, are said to stimulate the production of white blood cells which help in our fight against disease. Most pharmaceutical drugs tend to suppress symptoms rather than assist the body's innate healing mechanisms. Essential oils work more slowly, but when used correctly they assist the body in its healing process without the risk of side-effects.

When inhaled, aromatherapy oils are absorbed into the mucous membranes that line the nose. Olfactory cells connect directly with the brain, therefore the sense of smell has a powerful and immediate effect. Please remember that with all alternative therapies, remedies should be selected on a very individual basis. Please use your knowledge and intuition in carefully selecting the oils you use. Some oils will counteract the effects of homoeopathic remedies. If in doubt, contact a professional.

Dilution and contraindications

When diluting the oils, remember to use a 2–3% dilution. That is, 2–3 drops of essential oil per teaspoon of base oil. Use a 1% dilution for the face, or one drop of essential oil per teaspoon of base oil. Generally speaking, you should avoid using essential oils on children under two years old, although a couple of drops of a mild essential oil such as lavender or chamomile in 30 ml of almond oil is acceptable for sleeplessness, teething and tummy aches. Use 1% dilution on children aged between two and four, and 2% on children until the age of twelve. Afterwards the adult dilution can be used. Elderly or very frail people should use a 1% dilution.

There are many base oils, but the most common are almond and grapeseed oil, since they are fairly easy to purchase. They are also suitable for most skin types. They contain vitamins, minerals and proteins, and are gentle enough to use on the face.

Some of the most versatile essential oils include benzoin, bergamot, chamomile, eucalyptus, lavender, peppermint and ti-tree. All of the oils have many properties and a blend of two or three can often help with many problems at once.

Seven essential oils

Benzoin is made from tree gum and smells rather sweet, like vanilla. It comes from tropical countries in South East Asia and traditionally was used for driving away evil spirits. Benzoin is a grand remedy for stress and tension, since it helps one let go of worries and instils a feeling of confidence. It helps control blood sugar levels as well as respiratory disorders, and is very useful for dry, cracked skin. It has been used in cosmetics for centuries and is well known for its value in beauty treatments. It can make a person drowsy, so it is best avoided when concentration is needed.

Bergamot[3] is made from the peel of a citrus fruit and has a light, delicate aroma, rather like an orange. The oil takes its name from a small town in Italy, Bergamo, where the oil was originally cultivated. Bergamot is photosensitive and should be avoided if going outside into strong sunlight[4]. One drop can be applied neat to the skin to heal a cold sore or pimple, however, it is photosensitive and can irritate sensitive skin (a little white patch can appear on your skin if you go out into strong sunlight after it has been applied). Bergamot has a very uplifting nature. Research has shown that it benefits depression, anxiety and hysteria. It is very effective when dealing with infections, particularly cystitis, since it acts as a powerful disinfectant of the urinary tract.

Chamomile (or Camomile) is a very calming and relaxing oil and is often a first choice for children, particularly for stomach ache. It has a fruity, apple-like fragrance and is indigenous to Britain. German chamomile is deep blue in colour. Chamomile should be avoided in the first few months of pregnancy, but it is useful for regulating the menstrual cycle. It is a good oil for dull muscular pain and is particularly good for low back pain. It is also used for insomnia, nervous conditions and allergic reactions, including hay fever.

Eucalyptus is made from the Australian gum-tree, which can reach 300 feet. It is a very powerful essential oil, so much care should be taken with dosage. It should not be used by people with high blood pressure, since it could increase it further, or by epileptics. It can antidote homoeopathic remedies. It is well known for its beneficial action on the respiratory system, soothing inflammation and clearing mucus. It is a cooling oil both on the emotions and in easing fevers. It can be used in a massage or foot-bath to help relieve rheumatism.

Lavender is known as the queen of essential oils. It is made from the gently rounded lavender bush. It is calming and balancing, but it should be avoided by people with low blood pressure and pregnant women. For centuries lavender has been used in linen drawers to keep moths at bay, for cleansing wounds, for minor cases of epilepsy and for healing burns, cuts, stings and bruises. Rudolph Steiner maintains that lavender stabilises the Physical, Etheric and Astral bodies, which has a positive effect on the physical body. It can balance psychological disorders, has a sedative action on the heart, and is good for insomnia, sharp pain, respiratory disorders (asthma, coughs, colds and throat infections), menstrual problems and is valuable for most skin conditions. Lavender is one of the oils that may be applied neat[4] to the skin, but only one to two drops, since it is immediately absorbed by the skin and is passed into the circulatory system.

Peppermint was used by the ancient Egyptians, Greeks and Romans. It is a native of Europe. The best essential oil is from England since the herb favours damp conditions. Much care needs to be taken with dosage, since it can irritate sensitive skin and mucous membranes. It should be avoided by pregnant women and nursing mothers since it can discourage the flow of milk, as well as by anyone taking homoeopathic remedies as it may antidote them. Peppermint is well known for its action on the digestive system. It has a relaxing effect on the stomach muscles and is useful for vomiting, diarrhoea, constipation, flatulence, colic, nausea and travel sickness. It can help with headaches, but it is best to burn it for this problem. Peppermint can also help with numbness of the limbs.

Ti-tree (or Tea Tree) oil is produced in Australia only, where the Aborigines have long recognised the healing nature of the tree. Ti-tree is antibiotic, antiseptic, antiviral, anti-fungal and stimulating. Probably the most important effect of ti-tree oil is that it helps the immune system fight off infectious disease. It is also an expectorant (helps clear coughs and colds) and a good insecticide.

Three exercises

• To boost your immune system buy the essential oil that most appeals to you. Make a 2.5% dilution and use it in your bath or apply it directly to the skin. Visualise the energy of the plant penetrating every cell of your body. See the energy of this plant making you stronger.

• Instead of buying an insecticide for the garden, try using an environmentally friendly mixture of oil and water to spray on your fruits, vegetables and flowers. Use 4–8 drops of ti-tree essential oil in 4 litres of water, shake vigorously and spray when needed.

• Ants can be deterred by the essential oil of peppermint. They hate the smell and will go out of their way to avoid it. To clear a nest apply 1–2 drops of neat essential oil of peppermint and watch the exodus. If ants are coming into your house, place 1–2 drops wherever they enter. A peppermint plant often has the same effect.

Massage

In the 5th century B.C. Hippocrates said, 'A physician must be experienced in many things but assuredly also in rubbing – for things that have the same names have not always the same effect, for rubbing can bind a joint that is too loose and loosen a joint that is too tight; rubbing can bind and loosen; can make flesh or cause parts to waste; hard rubbing binds, soft rubbing loosens. Much rubbing causes parts to waste, moderate rubbing makes them grow.'[5]

When disease or injury occur, natural therapies can be used to stimulate the body's natural healing agents. There are many alternative approaches to holistic health, but one of the most basic tools for health maintenance is our need for touch. The Chinese used massage 5,000 years ago to prevent, ease and heal pain. The Hindus, Japanese, Egyptians, Greeks and Romans all used a form of massage as a part of their system of medicine. There is an instinctive need within us all to touch and be touched. Massage is an instinctive medicine which we all have at our command and it has both a psychological and physiological effect. The various movements stimulate the immune system while giving the patient a sense of wellbeing. Gentle touch expresses sympathy and caring while inducing relaxation and warmth which can help ease pain.

A full body massage will increase the venous and lymph flow, eliminate accumulated waste products, increase muscle contractility and tone, assist in the interchange of tissue fluids, help break down fat and improve body metabolism. It is also a decongestant and good for the skin. By means of relaxation, massage can also bring relief to insomnia and it can help ease headaches and migraines. Although massage cannot cure rheumatism and arthritis, it can ease the discomfort. Massage can bring great relief to tense muscles, particularly in cases of neck, shoulder and back pain. It can improve digestion, relieve bowel complaints and ease respiratory problems. When used in conjunction with aromatherapy, massage becomes a very effective tool for mind, body and spirit.

There is a strong link between stress and illness. Stress has been linked to high blood pressure and heart disease. After an emotionally stressful event, the body is less resistant to disease, so disorders such as headaches, backaches, acne and infertility are more likely to develop. Massage, the most ancient form of stress control, can enable the body, mind and spirit to relax and find harmony and balance once again.

Like all techniques, massage is not for everyone. Contraindications to massage include: cancer[6], areas of septic foci or pus (due to the risk of spreading the infection), areas of contagious or infectious skin conditions, pregnancy (great care must be taken with pregnant women), first three days of menstruation and cardiovascular conditions (including thrombosis, phlebitis, angina pectoris and hypertension). Avoid areas of varicose veins, unrecognised bumps and lumps, recent scar tissue (six months for major surgery and three months for minor) and areas of unexplained inflammation or pain. If in doubt, or if you are currently being treated for a medical condition, ask a professional for advice.

Anti-stress exercise for carers and health practitioners

Try the following self-massage exercise[6]. This method is particularly good for stress. It concentrates mainly on the neck, shoulders, face and head. Find a comfortable position either sitting or standing. Take your shoes off and loosen any constrictive clothing, particularly around the waist. Notice how you are feeling. Take a few deep breaths. Imagine you are breathing in feelings of peace and breathing out anxiety. You can remain sitting for this exercise.

1. Raise your shoulders to your ears as you inhale; pause for a moment, then drop your shoulders as you exhale.
2. Circle the point of your shoulder on each side; first on the right, then the left. Afterwards, circle the shoulders together clockwise, then anti-clockwise.
3. Move your head from side to side; front to back; ear to shoulder.
4. Rest your left hand on your waist. Lean to the right, taking your arm over your head. Stretch. Repeat on the other side.
5. Raise your arms above your head. Stretch. Interlock your hands and circle your trunk clockwise then anti-clockwise.
6. Move your eyes up/down; left/right; clockwise; anti-clockwise.
7. Pucker your lips, then relax. Open your mouth wide, then relax.
8. Holding your right elbow in your left hand, massage your left shoulder, squeezing the top of the shoulder with your right hand. Then do the other side.
9. Using both hands, finger massage the back of your neck.
10. Using your thumbs, press gently under the back of your skull.

11. Using your fingers, gently massage all over your face, forehead and ears. Do this with circular movements of the thumbs or fingers – this is known as 'petrissage'.

12. Rub scalp briskly and gently pull your hair.

13. Making your right hand into a fist, gently pound your neck, shoulders and upper back. Repeat with the left hand.(Make sure you are sitting down as you relax.)

14. Breathe out and allow yourself to sigh as you are doing this. Take a few moments to become aware of your body. Silence your mind and listen to the rhythm of your breathing.

15. Feel the chair you are sitting on. Feel your feet on the floor.

16. Wriggle your toes; stretch your legs and feet away from you.

17. Look down before looking up.

After doing this exercise a few times on yourself you might want to practice this technique on your friends and colleagues. There is no substitute for the quality of another person's touch.

---

[1] Ruler of Egypt from 1361 to 1352 B.C.

[2] Bergamot is photosensitive, so avoid strong sunlight after application.

[3] Bergamot is considered carcinogenic (cancer causing) so cancer patients should avoid it. Like other essential oils, care must be taken with dilution.

[4] Cancer patients should never use neat essential oils.

[5] W.E. Arnould-Taylor, *The Principles and Practice of Physical Therapy*, Cheltenham: Stanley Thornes, 1977, p. 97.

[6] Some people believe that massage can cause cancer to spread more rapidly throughout the lymphatic system. This is a controversial issue and you will have to make up your own mind. Once the cancer is terminal, then massage is only going to act as a type of pain relief. When someone is dying, touch is truly needed. Obviously the anti-stress exercise would not be appropriate, but instead gentle effleurage (stroking) and petrissage could be applied.

Books for further reading

Denise Brown, *Aromatherapy*, London: Headway, 1993.

Denise Brown, *Massage*, London: Headway ,1993.

Patricia Davis, *Aromatherapy An A-Z*, Saffron Walden: C.W. Daniel, 1988.

Patricia Davis, *Subtle Aromatherapy*, Saffron Walden: C.W. Daniel, 1992.

Nigel Dawes and Fiona Harrold, *Massage Cures: the family guide to curing common ailments with simple massage techniques*, London: Thorsons, 1990.

Wanda Sellar, *The Directory of Essential Oils*, Saffron Walden: C.W. Daniel, 1992.

Christine Wildwood, *Holistic Aromatherapy*, London: Thorsons, 1992.

Valerie Ann Worwood, *The Fragrant Pharmacy: a complete guide to aromatherapy and essential oils*, London: Bantam, 1993.

Useful addresses

International Federation of Aromatherapists, 46 Dalkeith Road, London SE21 8LS.

Northern Institute Of Massage, 100 Waterloo Road, Blackpool, Lancashire FY4 1AW.

West London School of Therapeutic Massage, 41 St Luke's Road, London W11 1DD.

I HAVE

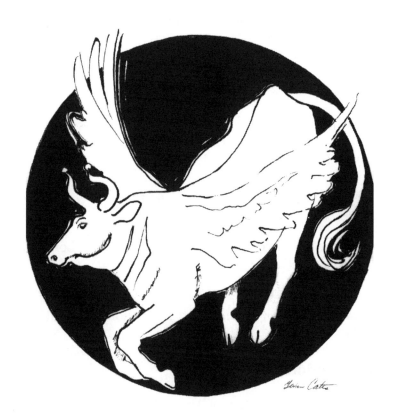

TAURUS
"Winged Bull"

II

Colour therapy and Aura-Soma

*The morning star is like a man; he is painted red
all over; that is the color of life.*
– A Pawnee priest.

Colour therapy is as old as recorded medicine. For a long time it was dismissed as superstition. Now physicists and mystics are coming together and realising the importance of energy work. The Tibetans say that a rock is only solidified sound. Physicists say that we live in a holographic universe, that we are merely particles and waves[1]. Both scientists and mystics are beginning to agree that we live in a universe that is alive and ever changing. We live in a world composed of colour and music.

Light and colour have always been part of our life on earth. Primitive people, or the original people, observed nature and used colour symbolically as a part of their society. The Ancient Egyptians used colour as part of their means of communication, particularly in hieroglyphics. Magicians wore blue breastplates to symbolise the sacredness of their judgements. Temples, talismans, charms and burial trappings were often colour related.

In Greece, Pallas Athena[2] was often depicted wearing a golden robe, the colour of the causal plane[3], as a symbolic connection to God. Buddha also wore gold or yellow, except when pondering on man, at which time he wore red. Confucius[4] is associated with yellow, the intellect. In ancient Egypt and China people wore red amulets, rings, etc. to prevent wounding and the flow of blood. Lord Jehovah[5] was often associated with blue. The holy grail was reputedly emerald green. Pythagoras[6] is said to have used colour, as well as music and poetry, to cure disease. In the 11th century, Avicenna[7] dressed his patients in red and maintained that the colour had amazing healing qualities. Paracelsus[8], known in the 16th century as a genius, suggested that colour and light were vital to human health. He attempted to direct medicine back towards the spiritual and taught that disease was caused by disharmony. He used invocations, music, colour, talismans, charms, herbs, divine elixirs, diet, bleeding and purging to cure his patients. He was hailed throughout Europe for his work.

In the 17th century Isaac Newton[9] developed today's fundamental understanding of colour by shining a beam of light through a prism where it dispersed into the spectrum of seven colours: red, orange, yellow, blue, green, indigo and violet. Newton concluded that these were the basic colours of the universe and that the source of all colour is white light.

Goethe[10] elaborated on this theory of colour. He believed that boundaries of light and darkness were necessary in order to create colour. Refraction in itself was not enough, it was the interplay of light and darkness at the edge of the prism that created the rainbow spectrum. Goethe also discovered an eighth invisible colour, referred to as magenta.

In physics, light or colour rays are recognised by their particular wavelength (or measurement in space) and frequency (or measurement in time). The higher the frequency of colour, the shorter the wavelength of colour. As the colours emerge from the prism, there is a consistent sequential order to the rainbow of colour. Each colour also has its own unique wavelength. Red has the longest wavelength in the visible colour spectrum and the lowest vibratory rate or frequency. Violet has the shortest wavelength and the highest vibratory rate.

Today, colour therapy is seen as a new dimension in holistic healing. Often colour is combined with sound therapy, flower remedies, homoeopathy and other types of vibrational therapies. Another useful combination is with meditation, visualisation and affirmations.

A confrontation with the dark can be seen as a confrontation with the light. Each colour contains an inherent balance, however, within the balance also lies a duality. This is an exercise designed to help you get in touch with your emotions through colour. This technique also requires using the right hemisphere of the brain. As babies, many people experienced such emotions as contentment, fear, anger, love or rejection. These initial emotions coloured the way we view life. However, since our society is highly verbal (the right hemisphere is 'mute', the left hemisphere governs speech), we often ignore emotions. This tends to damage our creative expression. We must be aware of what we feel in order to be able to interpret what is taking place in the core or central part of our being. This exercise will help you become aware of what you feel, which should then lead you to greater intellectual and emotional freedom.

Exercise

Make eight colour cards. The colours should be red, orange, yellow, green, blue, indigo or royal blue, violet and pink. You can use coloured paper or make your own cards using water-colours and white paper or cardboard. Keep these cards with you over the course of the week and write on the appropriate one when you experience a strong emotion. By the end of the week you will probably see the emergence of a dominant emotion/colour.

Emotional keywords

Red is related to the base chakra[11] and issues to do with physical survival (sex, food and money). In yogic philosophy, it is the seat of kundalini power and holds the promise of spiritual awakening. Red is the symbol of life, strength and vitality. The emotional keywords are love, generosity, sacrifice, passion, greed and anger. As you see, there are both positive and negative emotions associated with each colour. Red is also related to the Earth and gives us the basic energy for life. If you are feeling tired or spaced out, red socks will help! Write any of the keywords that you experience on the red card.

Orange is related to the second or sacral chakra and issues to do with relationships and sociability. It holds the promise of enlightenment and is the symbol of the Buddha. It is akin to feminine energy, the energy of creation. When balanced, it is the colour of joy and dance. Look for feelings related to friends and family to do with desire, joy, fulfilment, courage, trauma and shock. Orange is also related to detachment, dependency, co-dependency and letting go.

Yellow is associated with the third or solar plexus chakra. It has to do with fear and the ego. It is a very active centre in most people. It is a symbol of the mind and intellect. The emotional keywords are happiness, self-worth, detachment, confusion, stress and criticism. Yellow is related to the ego or the sense of self.

Green is associated with the fourth or heart chakra and when correctly awakened is expressed as harmony, love and good will. When it is out of balance, it can lead to an unhappy emotional life, jealousy, bitterness and resentment. Look for the emotions listed above in your life. Is your heart centre balanced? If not, use the green visualisation later in this section to help open this chakra. Green helps you make decisions, find your own space and brings you correct prosperity.

Blue is associated with the fifth or throat chakra. It is the creative centre, especially of the spoken word – blue is the colour of communication. The emotional keywords are truth, devotion, inspiration, introversion, withdrawal, separation and any issues to do with communication. You can visualise the colour blue to protect yourself. To do this, visualise yourself putting on a long blue cloak which reaches down to your feet, with a hood which you place over your head. Then close up the cloak with a full-length zip. As you fasten your cloak, state that you are now protected from any outside influence or negative energies.

Indigo/royal blue is associated with the sixth or brow chakra and is linked to mysticism at its most profound. When fully awakened it leads to psychic powers. It is the centre of idealism, dreams and imagination. In a state of imbalance it leads to self-pity. The emotional keywords are creative inspiration, psychic communication, intuition, depression and self-pity.

Violet is associated with the seventh or crown chakra which is the seat of higher consciousness. It is the colour of royalty and dignity. It is related to our connection with others and our desire (or lack of it) to be on earth. The emotional keywords are healing, self-respect (or lack of it), dignity, aloofness, loneliness and grief. It is also the colour of spiritual service, spiritual guidance and transformation.

Pink is related to the reproductive organs. Pink can also flow through an open heart centre. It is related to unconditional love, compassion, harmony and holy sound. The emotional keywords are love (or lack of it), acceptance, sharing, optimism, selflessness and caring. In most countries pink is related to the feminine aspect: the mother, the lover and the goddess.

If you find yourself experiencing a negative emotion, select the colour it is linked to and visualise yourself taking a bath in that colour. Tell yourself that you are now seeking balance and harmony. You will soon find that you will feel the more positive aspects associated with the colour. You may also want to think about the colour clothing you wear. What do your clothes say? If you are wearing all black, you may be rebelling or in a state of denial. If you want to attract more love into your life, wear pink!

Green visualisation[12]

Find a comfortable position, either sitting with your back against a wall or in a supine position[13], and make sure that you are warm. You may want a blanket or warm clothing. Relax. Take three deep breaths, sighing as you exhale. Imagine that your body stretches the length of the room and then comes back to normal. Then imagine yourself becoming as wide as the room, then back to normal. See your spirit self stand up and leave the body. Know that you are safe and can come back at any time.

Imagine that you are following a path through a forest. Observe the designs made by the leaves, vines and roots of the majestic old trees. Look up at their branches stretching towards the light of the heavens. Feel the dampness of the air. Listen to the sounds of the twigs snapping and the rustle of the leaves as you continue to walk along the path. All else is silent. The path leads through a natural archway created by trees. Only thin shafts of light are able to penetrate the green forest.

Look for your special tree. When you reach it, you find a comfortable mossy bank. Sit down with your back against the tree and become aware of the atmosphere. Talk to the tree in a loving and receptive way. Ask it to share its energy with you. Observe any colours that emanate from the tree. Feel the energy of the tree entering your body, travelling through your spine and energising the nerves, organs and cells. When you feel completely energised, thank the tree.

Now lie down and look up at the branches covered with leaves of various shades of green. Where the light filters through, the leaves take on a lighter colour than those in the shade. Try to sense and feel with your body the various shades of green. Which shade of green do you feel you need the most? As you inhale, visualise a shaft of this colour horizontally entering your heart chakra, removing any blockages which may be present. As you exhale, allow the colour to radiate out into your aura. Try to be aware of this colour bringing the positive and negative energies of your body into balance. When you are ready, bid the tree farewell and follow your path back through the archway of the forest. See yourself entering the meditation room and feel your spirit self slip back into your body. Feel the changes that have taken place. Increase your inhalation and exhalation as you become aware of your body once again.

Colour Therapies

Colour visualisation is a way of using the imagination to create the reality that you want. The idea is to acknowledge negative thought patterns and begin replacing them with positive thoughts. The wavelengths of colour support this process. Green, for instance, helps you find your direction and the way to bring prosperity into your life. To continue this process, visualise what you want in detail and see yourself possessing it. This puts you in a position of power. Another example would be visualising orange to help you become more gregarious. In addition you would visualise a successful social activity such as a dinner party.

Colour breathing revitalises our bodies. Hindus refer to the energy gathered through deep breathing exercises as prana, or the life force. In order to breathe deeply we need to be completely free of stress and tension. A rhythm is developed by concentrating on the in-breath and out-breath in a circular fashion. Exhaling as much as you can will help purify the body. This also awakens the solar-plexus, the power centre of the human. Colour breathing exercise involves breathing in the colours of each of the chakras (beginning with the magenta/crown) through all the chakras five times, each time seeing the colour becoming more pure. Another simple colour breathing exercise is consciously sending a colour you think a person might need to them on your out-breath.

Colour affirmations can help us transform negative belief systems into positive ones, and thus help us transform our lives. For instance: 'I, _____, am able to take responsibility for my thoughts, actions and health through the power and energy of the colour turquoise'[14].

Colourgenics is a way to recognise the messages people are sending by reading their clothing. The idea is that we surround ourselves with the colours that are visible reflections of our auras[15]. As our emotions change so do our colour choices. Colourgenics is about consciously interpreting these messages so we can live in greater harmony with others[16].

Aura-Soma

Aura-Soma colour therapy combines colour, crystal and herbal healing in more than ninety colourful balance bottles that glimmer like jewels in the sunlight. They were initially created by a blind English woman named Vicky Wall, through what she called 'divine inspiration'. Unlike most therapies, the bottle or remedy is selected intuitively by the patient. A therapist is needed to explain the potentials held within the bottle. The patient applies the oil and water mixture to the appropriate chakra area. Many feel that this is a true revelation in the healing process since it enables the patient to take responsibility for his/her healing process.

At the beginning of an Aura-Soma consultation, four balance oils are selected by the patient. The bottles are then 'read' by the therapist, who acts as a guide by explaining the potentials, blockages and future energies the patient is currently experiencing and drawing to him/herself. This therapy is particularly helpful for those working on developing their spiritual path.

[1] Reference: Michael Talbot, *The Holographic Universe*, New York: HarperCollins, 1991

[2] Pallas Athena, who sprung from the head of Zeus, is one of the most important Olympian deities in Greek mythology. The virgin warrior was the goddess of wisdom, war and peace, a guardian of cities (particularly Athens) and a patron of arts and crafts.

[3] The causal plane is related to the seventh level of the aura and is known as the mental level of the spiritual plane. See Section IV on Energy Therapies for explanation of the seventh level.

[4] A Chinese sage who lived in the 4th century B.C.

[5] God.

[6] A pre-Socratic Greek philosopher.

[7] The Persian physician, Ibn Sina (980–1037), was the most renowned philosopher of medieval Islam.

[8] Philippus Aureolus Paracelsus (1493–1541) was a Swiss physician and alchemist.

[9] Isaac Newton (1642–1727), the English physicist and mathematician, was considered by many to be the greatest scientist of all times.

[10] The writer and philosopher, Johann Wolfgang von Goethe (1747–1832), was one of the greatest figures of the German Romantic period.

[11] See Section IV on Energy Therapies for full explanation of chakras.

[12] Feel free to change the colour green to any other colour you would like to work with. Allow the tree to let you absorb the colour you need. See the appropriate colour(s) of light filtering through the leaves of the tree. See the colour you are working with radiating through your aura.

[13] Lying face upwards.

[14] The colour turquoise is very useful in building up the immune system. It also helps with inner difficulties, communication connected with the feelings and responsibility. It is the colour connected to the New Age, crystals, dolphins and mass media.

[15] See page 74 for full description of the aura

[16] See: Steven John Culbert, *The Body Language of Colour*, London: Foulsham, 1987.

Books for further reading

Reuben Amber, *Color Therapy: healing with color*, Santa Fe: Aurora Press, 1983.

Faber Birren, *Color Psychology and Color Therapy*, New Jersey: The Citadel Press, 1961.

Frank Don, *Colour Magic*, London: Aquarian, 1987.

Theo Gimbel, *The Colour Therapy Workbook: a guide to the use of colour for health and healing*, Shaftesbury: Element, 1993.

Roland Hunt, *The Seven Keys to Color Healing: diagnosis and treatment using colour*, San Francisco: Harper & Row, 1971.

Howard and Dorothy Sun, *Colour Your Life: discover your true personality through the colour reflection reading*, London: Piatkus, 1992.

Vicky Wall, *The Miracle of Colour Healing: Aura-Soma therapy as the mirror of the soul*, London: The Aquarian Press, 1990.

Pauline Wills, *The Reflexology and Colour Therapy Workbook: combining the healing benefits of two complementary therapies*, Shaftesbury: Element, 1992.

Useful addresses

Aura-Soma Colour Therapeutics, Dev Aura, Little London, nr Horncastle, Lincolnshire LN9 6QL.

Living Colour, 33 Lancaster Grove, Hampstead, London NW3 4EX.

I THINK

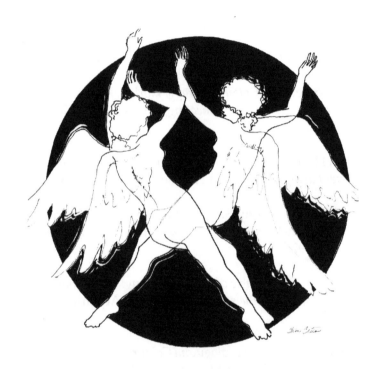

GEMINI
"Twin Angels"

III

The mineral kingdom:
a remembrance of crystal healing

Every cell thinks.
– Edison

Intelligence exists on all levels. Experiments have shown that plants respond to both love and abuse. Crystals also respond to the energy or attention they are given. Healers who are sensitive to the energies of crystals feel that when crystals are sent loving attention, they respond by offering, in turn, an endless supply of electromagnetic energy. The energy level of the healer increases and a spiritual quickening occurs, which leads to heightened consciousness. However, some say that manufactured crystals do not contain this life-force and do not offer the same natural assistance to the healer or visionary.

In astrology we learn that we are governed by four elements: fire, earth, air and water. Crystal healers take this a step further, suggesting that these elements are ensouled by beings called elementals which are activated by pure or unconditional love. The Native Americans discovered long ago that they could project thought patterns of love or hatred and release extremely powerful, and very different, frequencies of electromagnetic radiation, which was absorbed by all life-forms within a determined area.

The important point to understand is that crystals magnify the thoughts you project towards them. If you hold a crystal and think nothing, it is likely that you will feel nothing. On the other hand, if you genuinely wish to aid their evolutionary progress, they tend to respond. If you send them thoughts of unconditional love they respond in a loving way towards you.

Quartz crystals are energised by the moon. During the full moon the crystal is at its most powerful. When sleeping in the room with a quartz crystal during a full moon, some individuals have reported experiencing painful pressure in the head which is relieved when the crystal is removed. As the moon begins to wane, the crystal energy also begins to wane and there is a decrease in their outflow.

Crystals

Every individual has various behaviours and talents, rock crystals also have differing identities and qualities. The size of a crystal does not suggest its force. Edmund Harold suggests that like mankind each crystal contains an inherent, but inaudible, note or sound. The indwelling elemental, recognising an energetic relationship with you, draws you to it. The clear quartz crystals (referred to as positive or masculine crystals) often have a very clear and intense energy. These are the most popular of the crystals. They particularly help those who are confused by emotions. These clear quartz crystals help an individual discover a clearer or more focused outlook on life. They also raise or restore weakened energy levels.

Exercise: meditation with a crystal

Hold a crystal while listening to a piece of gentle music. Close your eyes and allow your mind to drift. Ask your crystal to show you the colours and shapes of the music. What did you see? Record it in your journal.

Other types of crystal

Cloudy or *milky quartz crystals* are referred to as feminine. They help to activate latent mediumistic qualities. They are very good for people who have trouble integrating the feminine or sensitive aspect of their nature. They help to ease headaches caused by tension. To try this, hold your feminine crystal in your right hand and point it to the area of pain or stress. Place your left hand on your throat or thyroid chakra (if it has to do with a power issue the abdomen or solar plexus chakra may be more appropriate). Close your eyes and concentrate on projecting love (some see this as pink light) to the elemental of the crystal. Within a short period of time the pain should begin to diminish. Ten minutes of this type of meditation should clear a painful headache entirely.

Crystal cluster formations contain very powerful energies. Clear or masculine clusters provide a good deal of stimulus for healers and therapists. Feminine clusters should be obtained when one is trying to develop spiritual or visionary talents. Clusters are designed to activate the crown chakra of anyone within its radius. For some people this can be a painful experience.

Smoky quartz is another powerful member of the mineral kingdom. It helps to release mental and emotional tensions, and dispels negative energy, allowing positive frequencies through. During healing sessions a smoky quartz crystal can be placed between the feet of the patient. (Should this result in pressure on the chakra points or cause palpitations of the heart, the crystal should be removed immediately.) Smoky quartz helps to keep a person centred while opening up emotionally. It also helps to dispel negativity.

Amethyst quartz clusters emit a powerful positive purifying energy. Used in a healing session, they have a positive effect upon the nervous system, can help skin disorders, are helpful for eye conditions, and help dispel negative or fearful thought patterns. Because of the purifying energy of amethyst clusters, they can be used to purify other rock crystals of negative vibrations they may have absorbed from a healing act. Simply leave the rock crystals on the amethyst cluster overnight and it will be revitalised, purified and ready to use in the morning. It is a good idea to clean your amethysts once a week in saline solution and rinse in warm water, so they will be able to continue their work for you.

Crystal balls are known as 'the mirror of the Seer', and have long been associated with the ability to reflect visions. When using a crystal ball, keep your eyes open. If you are gifted with second sight, you should begin to perceive other dimensions as you look into the crystal ball. If this does not happen, then you may find another type of crystal that can help you during meditation. In his book Crystal Healing, Edmund Harold indicates that crystal balls are related to the crystal mirrors once used in Atlantis by the temple virgins. Dr Raymond Moody takes this idea further in his book, Reunions: Visionary Encounters with Departed Loved Ones. Moody is one of the first modern medical doctors to investigate the paranormal and give it scientific legitimacy. He researched and built his own psychomanteum[1]. He later discovered that over half of his subjects saw or heard apparitions and that in all cases the visions were healing in a very positive way. People were able to see friends or relatives that they had worried about for years after sometimes painful or tragic deaths. In all cases the deceased looked younger, happier and seemed to be enjoying their lives on the other side. The seers are able to go back to their normal lives less afraid of death. Moody considers mirror gazing a type of self-exploration. It is possible to create your own psychomanteum. If you feel curious you may feel like experimenting with this technique.

Exercise: creating your own psychomanteum

To create your own psychomanteum you must first create the right atmosphere. Humour and the paranormal are connected. A feeling of playfulness helps facilitate visions, as does exercise. Ways of preparing yourself for mirror gazing would include walking in a beautiful forest or playing in the sea. It is important to relax. You could even listen to an audio tape of nature sounds. The second thing you do is to cover up or put away anything that reminds you of time. The dimension you are entering is not linear, so take off watches and cover up clocks. Looking at artwork, listening to music and reading books on esoteric subjects can also prepare you for an altered state. However, Moody found that the best way to prepare yourself is by looking at old photographs of the person or place you would like to visit, or by thinking of a question that really concerns you and focusing intently on it. Then take out your real quartz crystal ball. Allow your focus to become soft and your mind to wander. If you do not try too hard, you will begin to see images. When you have seen what is appropriate, the images will fade of their own accord.

If this is done in a light-hearted way, with a sense of playfulness, there is no danger involved. It is simply another way of seeing. If you are very interested in taking this technique further, read *Reunions*. Although no harm has ever come from this procedure, there are many superstitions surrounding these techniques. It is possible that old belief systems could cause problems. An intellectual understanding of the technique helps break through many outmoded religious beliefs. Humanity at large is beginning to realise that we each hold the keys that will unlock the answers to our many questions. There is no reason to seek outside of ourselves. There is no reason to be afraid.

Wearing crystals

It was recently alleged that wearing a crystal with its point downward depletes the human energy field. There are many views on this topic, but it is something to consider. Mike Booth, of Aura-Soma Colour Therapeutics, claims that to get optimum results from wearing members of the mineral kingdom, gems or crystals should be round in shape and form a complete circle around the neck. Edmund Harold suggests that one should select a double-terminated (or two-pointed) crystal to ensure an equal flow of energy. This type of crystal can also help someone suffering from a weak or impaired memory. Wearing crystals helps us to release repressed emotions. This is an important aspect of crystal healing as denied or repressed emotions can lead to serious illness. If you have worn a crystal all day, remember to purify it at night on an amethyst cluster – since a crystal saturated with negative vibrations can lead its wearer into a state of depression.

Exercise: six-pointed star

Crystals used in the six-pointed star formation correct both the physical and spiritual energy flow throughout the whole body. This exercise is best done with another person, one acting as healer and the other as recipient. Find eight crystals (or rocks) to use for this exercise. Use a clear quartz crystal for the generator. Sit down on the floor in lotus position if possible. If the recipient has a physical ailment, the largest crystal should be placed in front of the feet. If the person is in generally good health, however, the largest crystal should be placed at their back in alignment with their spine. The sequence should be as seen in the diagram. The sitting person is encircled with crystals: 1 at the back balances the spiritual side of the being; 2 and 5 on the left side relate to the lower half of

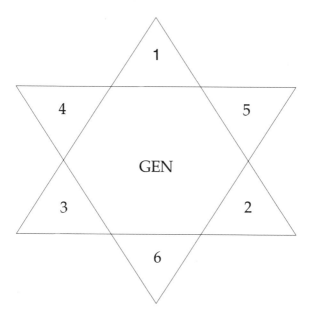

the physical and spiritual body; 3 and 4 on the right side of the body relate to the upper half of the body, both physically and spiritually. Crystal 6 balances the physical side of the being. The clear quartz 'generator' is held in the hands of the person receiving healing. It serves as the receptor for the energies being dispersed to the surrounding crystals. It unifies the force-field and allows the body to draw what it needs from this flow.

Beginning with crystal 1, place the crystals in numerical order around the recipient. This sets up the correct energy field. Crystals 1, 2 and 3 form the spiritual trinity, while 4, 5 and 6 form the physical trinity. This helps to repolarise and balance the vibrations within the person. The healer then uses an additional crystal, called the control crystal, and passes it in a circular motion around the person. This connects the energies of the six crystals. The healer completes twelve circles and then allows the recipient to rest within the star formation for ten minutes. To achieve a permanent effect, this exercise should be performed once weekly for four weeks.

The Ascended Masters

As we enter the New Age there is an increasing amount of talk about Ascended Masters. These are beings of goodness and light who have incarnated many times upon the earth in an attempt to perfect themselves. Having mastered their base emotions, they are now part of a spiritual hierarchy responsible for the growth and development of this planet. Their task is to reactivate conscious awareness of the true or higher Self. They are helping humanity undergo a change in consciousness from third dimensional reality – which has to do with power, fear and ego – to the fourth dimensional reality, or the spiritual plane. One of their tasks is to reacquaint humanity with the ancient knowledge of colour, sound and the mineral kingdom.

The names of these Masters were received psychically by Madame Blavatsky[2], Annie Besant[3], Alice Bailey[4], Vicky Wall[5] and Mike Booth[6], among others. The Masters are not demigods, but beings of light that act as a bridge to God/Goddess/All That Is. Sensitives state that there is more help on this planet than there has ever been in the history of earth. In the past the rays connected to these Masters shone separately, now they are working collectively. They are here to assist the awakening of the planet and are available to the souls who want to be part of the divine plan.

The Lord or eldest of all the Masters is known as *Maha* (meaning greater) *Chohan* (teacher). He has never incarnated in physical form but was known as the Lord of civilisation in Lemuria. He is connected to native American teaching, particularly the Racoon (crazy wisdom).

Maha Chohan is linked to aquamarine, the stone that carries a lot of energies and the promise of the incoming new aeon. He teaches us to take responsibility for ourselves and is never amused when we try to play God (i.e. genetic engineering) or abuse animals. He assists us in communicating with the being within. This work can be intensified with awareness of the mineral kingdom.

At this time there are seven Ascended Masters. The essence of *El Morya* helps us find our life purpose on the earth plane. He helps open the door to communication from above. His female counterpart, *Lady Miriam*, is represented by our pale blue globe. She contains the nurturing energy of the Mother as she shields and protects the organic layer of the earth. These beings help us understand that we are part of God/Goddess/All That Is. Gem correspondences include sapphire and lapis lazuli.

Kuthumi symbolises the light. He helps cut through confusion so that we may find clarity within. He connects the three kingdoms (devic, human and angelic) and facilitates communication between them. He is also intimately connected with the energy of numbers. Another name for Kuthumi is the Maitreya Buddha, or the future Buddha. Kuthumi sits in the future projecting love and understanding into the present. Gem correspondences include citrine.

Lady Nada is known as the consort of Christ. She encourages us to look inside for unconditional love and acceptance. She helps us suspend self-judgement and clear negativity. If we set up unconditional love in our aura, then we are much more likely to attract it into our lives. Her vibration works well with rose quartz.

The essence of *Hilarion* helps us step into the possible self. He teaches the way, the truth and the light; he helps you find your own truth. He brings in new direction and new space. His energy penetrates the heart centre and helps us face deep emotional issues. When we work with Hilarion we learn to trust ourselves. Gem correspondences include the emerald and green calcite.

Serpais Bey is the pure light that contains all colours. He represents a new dimension and a new beginning. His energy is entirely sympathetic with quartz crystal. He is helping us move away from carbon (coal and oil), which pollutes the earth, towards silica (crystals, microwaves, digital watches) as a healthy energy source.

The Christ, or Christ consciousness, helps us with the acceptance of self at the deepest level and thus offers the promise of awakening the true, enlightened Self. The Christ is a very protective energy. He reveals the full power of the light as we move into another dimension. At some point the little self has to be sacrificed so the greater Self can flourish. The Christ also helps with forgiveness and reconciliation. The gem correspondences are the red stones: ruby and garnet. The ruby helps to balance the base chakra; it helps us with the material side of life, is grounding, yet awakening, and can help balance all the other chakras. It is generally necessary to wear a complete necklace in a rounded bead form to effectively enter the auric field.

St Germain[7] is known as the Master of transmutation. His violet ray overshadowed Shakespeare who gave esoteric information in the form of drama to the masses. St Germain teaches that if you make each step with love and care, then when you arrive, there will be loving and caring. His energy is closely linked to the amethyst.

To get in touch with these master energies, select a gem or crystal and sit quietly with it. Ask to feel the energy of a particular Master and carefully observe the sensations in your body. You may see the glimmer of a face or hear a faint whisper that could easily be music.

Another way to explore the energies is to use the Aura-Soma Quintessences[8]. There are fourteen Quintessences, each linked to a different Master. Vicky Wall described them as the Source of Light beyond stillness. The colours help you to recognise your personal Master and achieve direct contact via higher consciousness.

[1] A place where spirits of the dead are summoned as a means of divination so that they can be asked questions about future or other hidden things. Dr Moody's psychomanteum is aimed at healing bereavement rather than divination.

[2] Helena Petrova Blavatsky (1831–1891) was a Russian spiritualist, author and co-founder of the Theosophical Society. Her most important work is *The Secret Doctrines*.

[3] Annie Besant, born in London in 1847, was a social reformer and theosophist. She became president of the Theosophical Society in 1907 and continued until her death in 1933. She wrote numerous books and articles on theosophical belief that are still considered some of the best work on the subject.

[4] Alice Bailey channelled the Tibetan Master DK, or Djwal Khul, while he was still in earthly incarnation. This resulted in an illuminating series of books on the occult.

[5] Vicky Wall was the founder of Aura-Soma Colour Therapeutics. See Colour Therapy, Section II, for more details.

[6] Mike Booth, teacher and clairvoyant, is now the head of Aura-Soma Colour Therapeutics in Lincolnshire.

[7] Also known as Master Ragoczy.

[8] See Colour Therapy.

Books for further reading

Dr Frank Alper, *Exploring Atlantis*, California: Quantum, 1981.

Edmund Harold, *Crystal Healing: a practical guide to healing with quartz crystal*, London: Aquarian, 1990.

Melody, *Love is in the Earth – A Kaleidoscope of Crystals: the reference book describing the metaphysical properties of the mineral kingdom*, Colorado: Earth-Love Publishing House, 1991.

Raymond Moody, *Reunions: visionary encounters with departed loved ones*, New York: Villard Books, 1993.

John D. Rea, *Patterns of the Whole: healing and quartz crystals: a journey with our souls*, Colorado: Two Trees Publishing, 1986.

Michael J. Roads, *Journey into Oneness: a spiritual odyssey*, California: Kramer, 1994.

To obtain crystals or for crystal workshops

John W. Scott, B.M. Box 1431, London WC1N 3XX. Tel: (01539) 729069. Fax: (01539) 729069.

For more information about psychomanteums

Dr Raymond A. Moody, Theatre of the Mind, Anniston, Alabama, U.S.A.

I FEEL

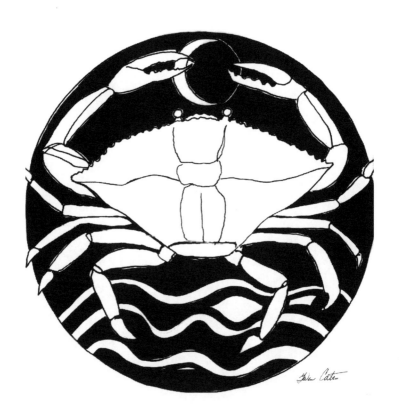

CANCER
"The Crab and Crescent Moon"

IV

Energy therapies

Intuition is always a step ahead of science.
– Bachler

Dowsing and pendulums

Emperor Yu wrote the first book about dowsing and the dowsing rod in 2,000 BC. In ancient China, before a house was built the site had to be examined by a dowser. Dowsing, either with rods or a pendulum, is an ancient technique used throughout all the countries of the world. The various types of rods include the simple forked twig, metal loops and bent wires. There are also numerous types of pendulums. The basic pendulum is simply a string or a chain with a heavy object on the end, such as a copper bolt or a crystal. These instruments have been used throughout the ages to detect water for wells, harmful radiation and electricity.

In order to dowse effectively a person must train him or herself to dedicate his or her energy and talent toward the good of humanity. Intent is an important element behind successful dowsing. The church even agrees to this: 'If ... a Christian wants to do God's will and protects himself with prayers when doing radiaesthesic works.and uses his or her instruments only in a helping way, based on love, when examining houses and finding water, then this work is blessed by the Church (Decree of 26 March 1942)'[1].

Exercise: using a pendulum

Most people can dowse. Try it! Find a piece of string and a bolt or a button to weight the string down with. Put the bolt or button on the string. Hold the string between your index finger and your thumb. Keep your arm relaxed and your wrist slightly bent. You want to keep your energy flowing and your mind completely clear of thoughts. Ask the pendulum to show you which way is 'yes'. The answer it gives you will be your answer. There is no correct way. The possibilities include a clockwise or counter clockwise swinging or a line swinging left to right or up and back. Then thank the pendulum and ask it to show you the movement for 'no'. It will give you another answer. Generally, my pendulum swings clockwise for 'yes' and counter clockwise for 'no'. There are times when it answers another way, so it is good idea to check 'yes' and 'no' every time you begin asking questions.

Once you have mastered the basics you can then test for energies. Hold your pendulum over your palm and see if it picks up the energy of the minor chakra in the centre of your palm. See which way it spins.

Now that you have the pendulum going, as long as the intent is correct, you can test for anything. Try asking it about general health problems, such as vitamin and mineral imbalances. Don't complicate the issue. Simply dowse over pages 11–14 of this workbook asking to find a healthy nutritional balance for your body. Say something like: 'At this given point in time do I need vitamin C? Yes or no.' Make sure you are very clear when you ask questions. This is where beginning dowsers often go wrong. Ask if you need vitamin C at this point in time, not sometime during the course of your life. It is better if you do not look at the pendulum since you do not want to influence the answers. Also it is a waste of time asking the pendulum what is going to happen in the future. The future is up to you. You are creating your future. The pendulum cannot predict what you are going to do. You may want to ask: 'Would it be good for me to visit dad today?' You won't know exactly what 'good' means, but at least if you go you will be acting to benefit both of you. Ask questions that will help keep your body in harmony and balance with the universe. When you begin to listen to the pendulum, to your Self, you will find that your ability to 'link into' or be more connected to all things is greatly strengthened. Many people have used dowsing, muscle resistance testing or kinesiology to cure themselves of serious illnesses. This does not always happen, and there is no proof to begin to substantiate the claim, but there are many people who will tell you stories of their illnesses disappearing as soon as they got in touch with their Self.

Chakras

Chakras are a 4,000 year old Indian system of describing the subtle bodies of humankind. They are known as the energy centres in the body. The word chakra is Sanskrit, meaning 'wheel' and it conveys not only the idea of a circle but also of turning. It is said that the chakras constantly revolve. There are many chakras situated throughout the body; generally, healers work on the seven major chakras situated on the midline of the body.

The chakras are often described as running along the spine. However, each chakra should be thought of as extending right through the body from front to back. The energy of each chakra extends well beyond the visible body of matter into the aura[2]. Each layer of the aura is associated with a chakra. The chart on page 72 helps to illustrate the location and function of the major chakras.

The root or base chakra is related to the colour red. It is located at the base of the spine or the perineum and is linked to the sexual and reproductive system (the testes and vagina), as well as to the tailbone, legs and feet. It is associated with survival, grounding, physical needs, safety and sexuality.

The sacral chakra is related to the colour orange.

Chakra	Location	Connection
base	gonads	physical functioning and physical sensation feeling physical pain or pleasure
sacral	below navel	emotions — emotional life and feelings
solar plexus	above navel	mental life, linear thinking
heart chakra	heart (midline)	love for mate and humanity
throat chakra	throat	related to divine will, power of the word, communication, taking responsibility for actions
third eye	forehead	celestial love
crown	above head	higher mind, integration of spiritual and physical make-up

It is located below the navel and is linked to the spleen, ovaries, adrenal gland, uterus, kidneys and urinary tract. It is associated with our emotional needs, attachments, pleasure and addictions.

The solar plexus chakra is related to the colour yellow. It is located just above the navel and is linked to the pancreas, stomach, liver, small intestine and the digestive system. It is associated with mental energy, will power, joy, fear, the ego and self-criticism.

The heart chakra is associated with the colour green. It is located in the centre of the chest and is linked to the heart, thymus, lungs and breathing. It is associated with harmony, balance, new ideas, growth, receiving and giving.

The throat chakra is associated with the colour blue. It is located on the mid-throat and is linked to the thyroid, parathyroid, neck, colds and sinus conditions. It is associated with communication, creativity, speaking and releasing.

The brow or third eye chakra is associated with the colour indigo. It is linked to the pituitary and hypothalamus glands[3], the eyes and the autonomic nervous system. It is associated with dreams, psychic communication, depression, detachment and the imagination.

The crown chakra is associated with the colour violet. It is also sometimes referred to as the third eye. It is associated with spiritual guidance, self-respect, dignity, aloofness, isolation and grief.

Additionally, you may choose to work with an eight or above crown chakra, associated with the colour magenta. It is linked to the pineal gland and the central nervous system. It is associated with compassion, gentleness, non-attachment, spiritual healing and celestial love.

Exercise: feeling the chakras

Ask a friend who is open to experimentation to lie down on the floor. Take out your pendulum and hold it about three inches above the body. Beginning at the top of the thighs, move the pendulum slowly up over the pelvic area until you can feel the energy of the base chakra. It is likely that your pendulum will begin to swing in a clockwise manner. Take note if it swings in an oval shape or a counter clockwise direction. If so, ask your friend to visualise a circular red plate spinning in a clockwise direction.

Continue to feel each chakra as you move up the body. If the second chakra, or any other, is spinning in a counter clockwise position that may be normal for the person. Generally, a woman on her menstrual cycle will have a counter clockwise spin to her second chakra. Don't try to alter anything; just feel the energy and have your friend continue to visualise the appropriate colour for each spiralling chakra.

After feeling the above crown chakra ask your friend to visualise each chakra shutting down. Begin with the eighth and work down to the first chakra. A good way to do this is to visualise a flower closing for the night, first a magenta flower, then a violet flower, then an indigo flower and so on. This heals and protects the energy centres.

The aura

The aura of the average human extends from the body about a metre. It appears as moving colour swirling around the physical body. In the 1950s, Kirlian photography[4] made auric sight available to everyone, including its flaws which often are an early indication of a developing disease. Humans, animals and plants have auras, that is, an energy-field that surrounds the body. In artwork depicting religious masters we often see the halo surrounding the head as a symbol of their spiritual attainment. Navajo rock paintings sometimes show a glow around a person. The aura can also be seen in Persian, Japanese and Indian artwork. Some healers describe the aura as a subtle body, or a series of subtle bodies.

The first layer of the human aura is known as the *etheric body*. 'Etheric' comes from the word 'ether': the state between energy and matter. Generally, the etheric can be seen or felt about a quarter of an inch away from the skin. It has the same structure as the physical body, only it is made up of tiny webs of light. The second auric layer is known as the *emotional body* and is associated with feelings. It roughly follows the outline of the physical body, but is much more fluid than the etheric. It extends one to three inches from the body. The third auric layer is known as the *mental body*. It extends beyond the emotional body and tends to expand or become brighter when the person is focusing on a mental task. A colour aura photograph can be taken at health fairs. This shows your current emotional and mental state. If you have another photograph taken the following week it is likely that other colours will be present.

These three inner auric layers have to do with work in the physical world. The three outer auric layers, and beyond, are more closely associated with the spiritual world. The fourth layer or *astral body* is associated with the heart chakra and generally extends six to twelve inches from the physical body. The heart centre is the link between the physical and spiritual worlds. The astral body is associated with love and is the gateway to other realities.

The next layers are very ethereal and are seen or felt by only a few talented healers. There is no proof of their existence. However, Vicky Wall, Mike Booth, Barbara Brennan and others, continue to speak of the importance of these outer layers. The fifth layer is said to look like the negative of a photograph. It is here that we find the blueprint of our physical form. The sixth is associated with spiritual ecstasy which can be reached through meditation. When we begin to see light and love in everything, to understand our interconnectedness with all things and to feel, that we are one with God/Goddess/All that is, then we have raised our consciousness to the sixth layer. The seventh level or outer aura contains all the auric bodies associated with our present incarnation. Many of us that are experiencing a healing crisis of some sort will have a tree or mushroom-shaped aura. An advanced soul will have an egg-shaped aura which will contain all the colours of the rainbow.

Exercise: feeling the aura

With a little practice, most people can feel or see the first auric layer that surrounds the body. Hold your palms about two to five inches apart. Slowly move your hands away from each other, then begin to decrease and increase the space between them. Feel yourself building a ball of energy between your hands. Can you feel it? Try this with a friend. Is the energy ball between you stronger or weaker?

Now, take your hands eight to ten inches apart. Then slowly bring them back together until you feel a pressure pushing your hands out so that you have to use just a slight amount of force to bring your hands together. You have just felt your etheric body.

Take your hands apart again and begin to draw energy circles on your palms (keep the fingertip about an inch away from the palm). Can you feel anything? Try drawing circles on the palm or cheek of a friend.

Dim the lights in the room. Hold your hands up in front of you against a blank white wall pointing the fingertips together. Relax your focus and softly gaze at the space between your fingertips (keep them about one and a half inches apart). Make sure you do not look into bright light. Relax. What do you see? Move your hands closer and then further apart. Can you see a thin bluish-white film or web between your fingers? When you pull your hands apart the etheric layer sticks together like chewing gum. Experiment with this. How far can you pull the web before it separates?

Next time you have a bath look into the steamy mirror. Can you see your aura? Look to the left, but not straight on. Allow your focus to blur slightly. What colours do you see? You may want to draw it.

Kirlian photography

Throughout history many people have claimed to see auras. Discharges of energy, usually seen as a bluish light, have been seen and recorded since the beginning of history. A Russian research couple, the Kirlians, have made the aura visible to everyone with a technique known as Kirlian photography. This unconventional photographic process has existed since the late 1890s. Acupuncturists have been describing ch'i for nearly five thousand years. Kirlian photography is making ch'i visible to everyone.

Kirlian photography is a nonconventional photographic process in which photographs are produced from the action of high-frequency currents. The Kirlians wrote, 'The principle is based on the transformation of nonelectrical properties of the photographed subject into electrical ones, via motion of a field involving the controlled transfer of a charge from an object to a photographic screen.'[5]

Having a Kirlian photograph taken of your hand is a simple process. You go into a darkroom, remove all of your jewellery (so that it does not effect your energy), place your hand on some photographic paper resting on the Kirlian plate. Then you feel a brief electrical buzz while the photograph is being taken. The photographer then develops the image. Afterwards you take your photograph to someone who is trained in 'reading' the image.

Some massage practitioners will take a Kirlian photograph before and after your treatment so that you can see what sort of effect the massage has had on your body. What you hope to see is an increase in your vital force.

The photographs are generally read in a holistic way. The photograph is read in a way similar to the approach reflexologists use when examining the zones of the feet. By examining the dark outline of the palm the reader can see signs that relate to the health of your organs and skeletal system. Most therapists link physical and emotional problems. It is likely that the reader will suggest various colours, flower remedies and visualisations to you. Some people can also read a person's healing capacity and state of spiritual awareness.

Kirlian photography is offered at many mind–body–spirit fairs. Private workshops are run throughout Britain and can usually be found via your local yoga group.

Meridians

Ch'i is the Chinese name for the life-force or subtle energy that permeates the Universe and sustains all living things. The Chinese maintain that we bring a store of ch'i with us from the time of birth into physical existence. This is known as 'Before Heaven Ch'i'. During life more ch'i may be acquired via the breath, food, specific ch'i exercises and spiritual practices. This is known as 'After Heaven Ch'i'. Ch'i is distributed throughout our bodies via the meridians, of which there are twelve. Each meridian is connected with a particular organ or system of the body. The Chinese tend to relate emotions to the organs as well. The liver, for example, relates as much to anger as to the actual organ. The meridians function in pairs, with each pair being made up of one Yin and one Yang meridian. Ch'i moves from the head towards the feet through the Yang meridians on the back of the body. Yin meridians move from feet to head on the front of the body.

It takes quite a lot of practice to learn the meridians and even more experience to know whether they are in balance. Shiatsu therapists and acupuncturists specialise in this field. If you are interested contact a local practitioner.

Earth energies

Many doctors in Germany, Austria and France are known to use dowsers (people sensitive to the energies of the earth) as part of their health care programmes. In *Earth Radiation*, Kathe Bachler has put together some startling information on more than 3000 apartment houses and work places. She concentrates on the effect earth radiation has on human beings. She claims that she has found a significant link between geopathic stress and cancer, in fact, with illness of all kinds. Bachler writes:

> *Physicists tell us that the globe is surrounded by its own field of rays, waves, and energy, the so called earth field or earth magnetic field. These are natural, harmonious, good rays, and we need them to sustain life. However, at certain locations, plains, strips or zones, we find these fields of rays to be disturbed or dislocated. There we find disharmonious, harmful rays. These interfering rays are often called 'earth rays'. The areas where these earth rays are found we will call 'zones of disturbance' or 'areas of irritation'. Their causes can be subterranean or*

> *underground water courses, geological cracks or faults,*
> *hollow spaces, etc., or 'global grids', which have been re-*
> *discovered within the past few decades. These have become*
> *more recognised because their effect intensity have*
> *increased since our environment – especially our houses*
> *– have become so invaded by 'technical' and artificial rays.*

Studies have shown that sleeping on areas that are radiated makes it much more difficult for people to recover from disease. People sleeping on areas free of radiation generally respond to treatment much more rapidly. Bachler found that 95% of the time, chronically and severely ill people were either sleeping or working on places dominated by water currents and negative earth energies. When dowsing your house (or having some one do it for you) limit yourself to nets, grids and water currents. Simply look for the best places to sleep.

Bachler reminds us not to be alarmed, but rather be happy that there are energies in every room that can help us thrive or make us ill. We must learn to pay attention to the way the body is affected by its surroundings. What we should look for are the areas between the negative zones, since these are helpful and harmonious rays which are well suited for sleeping and working. To practise this, try the following exercise.

Exercise: energy location test

Standing quietly, or sitting on a wooden chair, examine the whole room slowly. In a relaxed and carefree manner, listen to your body. Move a few feet at a time. How do you feel? Take mental notes. When you are on a harmonious area, you feel well and will easily be able to remain there for ten minutes or so. However, when you feel uncomfortable or cannot breathe well then you are on a negative earth energy. Other signs will be feeling unwell, a tingling sensation, pulling cramps, pains in the region of the heart, or other pains.

Do this test in your bedroom. You only need about two square metres for a 6 x 3 ft bed. It is likely that you will easily find a healthful location in your room. In this way everyone can help him/herself without the aid of a dowser.

Most people do not need to sleep or work in a place completely free of radiation, however, if you are ill it becomes more important. You want to make sure that you are giving yourself the best chance to recover. Bachler has found that minor influences from zones of disturbance are usually tolerable, and reminds us that a healthful and peaceful lifestyle will counteract whatever damage might ensue from earth radiations.

[1] A note from the Archbishop of Salzburg, Dr Karl Berg. Reference: Kathe Bachler, *Earth Radiation*, Manchester: Wordmasters, 1989, p. xiv.

[2] See later in this section for full description of the aura.

[3] Many healers link the brow chakra to the pineal gland.

[4] See later in this section for full details.

[5] Stanley Krippner and Daniel Rubin (eds), *The Kirlian Aura: photographing the galaxies of life*, New York: Anchor Books, 1974, p. 35.

Useful books

Kathe Bachler, *Earth Radiation: the startling discoveries of a dowser, results of research on more than 3000 apartments, houses and work places*, Manchester: Wordmasters, 1989.

Barbara Ann Brennan, *Hands of Light*, London: Bantam, 1987.

Jane Downer, *Shiatsu*, London: Headway, 1992.

Michio Kushi, *How to See Your Health: book of oriental diagnosis*, New York: Japan Publications, 1980.

Stanley Krippner and Daniel Rubin (editors), *The Kirlian Aura: photographing the galaxies of life*, New York: Anchor Books, 1974.

Gustav Freiherr von Pohl, *Earth Currents: causative factor of cancer and other diseases*, Stuttgart: Frech-Verlag, 1983.

Useful pamphlet

Kathe Bachler, *'Noxious Earth Energies and Their Influence on Human Beings' Lecture*, 2nd June 1987. Translated by Ilse and Aubrey Pope, Essex.

Useful addresses

British Acupuncture Association and Register, 34 Alderney Street, London SW1V 4EV.

Council for Acupuncture, Suite 1, 19a Cavendish Square, London W1M 9AD.

International Register of Oriental Medicine, Green Hedges House, Green Hedges Avenue, East Grinstead, East Sussex RH19 1DZ.

I WILL

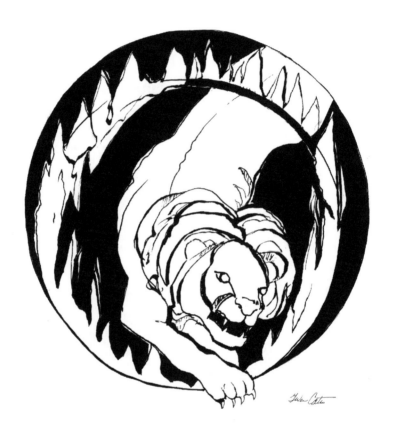

LEO
"The Fiery Hoop"

V

The gift of flowers:
the Bach flower remedies

To see the world in a grain of sand,
And heaven in a wild flower,
Hold infinity in the palm of your hand,
And eternity in an hour.
– William Blake

One of the best ways to begin to contact the love within ourselves is to go into the garden early in the morning and watch the flowers. When we listen to the birds singing, observe a small child or watch an act of generosity with an open heart, we begin to contact gratitude, love and beauty. When emotional or physical pain has become too much for us to bear, the best escape is to look at a beautiful flower.

A CONTEMPLATION UPON FLOWERS

Brave flowers, that I could gallant it like you,
And be as little vain;
You come abroad and make a harmless show,
And to your beds of earth again;
You are not proud, you know your birth,
For your embroidered garments are from earth.

You do obey your months and times, but I
Would have it ever spring;
My fate would know no winter, never die,
Nor think of such a thing;
Oh that I could my bed of earth but view,
And smile and look as cheerfully as you.

Henry King   *(1592-1669)*

Throughout history, people have connected healing and love with flowers. Remember Perdita's words[1]
from *The Winter's Tale*:

> .... *daffodils,*
> *That come before the swallow dares, and take*
> *The winds of March with beauty; violets dim,*
> *But sweeter than the lids of Juno's eyes*
> *Or Cytherea's breath; pale primroses*
> *That die unmarried ere they can behold*
> *Bright Phoebus in his strength — a malady*
> *Most incident to maids ....*

When a flower blossoms, it gives its beauty freely
and spontaneously to the world. Human beings generally try to get some advantage out of their beauty, clev-
erness or skills. Imagine a world where everyone gave
freely of their beauty and inherent gifts ....

Bach flower therapy

Over fifty years ago a Harley Street physician, Dr Edward
Bach, discovered a form of healing with wild flowers now
called Bach (pronounced Batch) flower remedies. There
are thirty-eight in total. This is a form of therapy that is
safe to use, even for people who are not trained in medicine. Bach flower remedies are used to treat or prevent psychological and physical illness and can be used alongside
other therapies. Bach wrote, 'Disease is solely and purely
corrective; it is neither vindictive nor cruel, but it is the
means adopted by our own souls to point to us our faults,
to prevent our making greater errors, to hinder us from
doing more harm, and to bring us back to the path of Truth
and Light from which we should never have strayed.'[2]
Dr Bach had a vision of a holistic approach to well-
being based on the concept of the perfect unity of all

things. He believed that every symptom of body, mind or spirit was a message to us, and that our task is to acknowledge and interpret these messages. Bach did not diagnose physical symptoms but instead concentrated on states of disharmony in the soul such as negative feelings or emotions. Bach remedies help us to balance the vital energies of our true nature, dissolving blockages and returning a negative to a positive state. We all have everything we need to be healthy, sometimes it has just shifted out of balance.

Edward Bach believed that each person should 'heal thyself'. It was his vision that these remedies be made available to all of mankind – doctors and lay people alike. They are designed for people who are working on their mental and spiritual growth. These are energetic remedies which act at more subtle levels influencing us via our energy system. This type of therapy also invites us to become more perceptive and to become much more aware of the intuitive/feminine side of our being.

In 1934 Bach wrote the following about the way his remedies work:

> *The action of these remedies is to raise our vibrations and open up our channels for the reception to the Spiritual Self; to flood our natures with the particular virtue we need, and wash out from us the fault that is causing harm. They are able, like beautiful music or any glorious uplifting thing which gives us inspiration, to raise our very natures, and bring us nearer to our souls and by that very act to bring us peace and relieve our sufferings. They cure, not by attacking the disease, but by flooding our bodies with the beautiful vibrations of our Higher Nature, in the presence of which, disease melts away as snow in the sunshine.[3]*

Bach believed that every person has a specific energy potential that he/she incarnates onto earth to fulfil. Each of us is part of the great plan of creation, and each of us has an immortal soul or true self, as well as a mortal personality that is presently on earth. Bach felt that there was a higher self that acted as a mediator between the immortal soul and the personality, and that each person unconsciously desires to live in harmony. However, Bach felt that to do this, the ideal qualities of the higher self had to be developed: gentleness, firmness, courage, constancy, wisdom, joyfulness and purposefulness. The flower remedies aid the development of these ideals. Bach felt that pride, cruelty, hatred, self-love, ignorance and greed were the true causes of disease. His idea was that if each personality would act harmoniously with its soul, then humankind would be able to live in perfect harmony.

Bach felt that two basic errors were the cause of disease. The first error he described as the personality not acting in accordance with its soul and having the illusion of being separate from it. When this is the case, the personality begins to wither and eventually dies, since the love that flows from the soul into the personality is the source of life.

The second error he described as the personality acting against the intentions of its higher self and soul. Bach felt that each one of us should freely develop our own lives according to the dictates of the soul alone.

The remedies therefore are designed to work effectively against negative soul states that eventually lead to physical illness. The flower remedies are designed to flood us with a higher harmonious energy so that negative states dissolve. The idea behind this is that the human soul contains all thirty-eight qualities of the Bach Flowers as energy potentials. The energy in the remedies helps the personality to re-establish contact and harmony with the soul[4].

Some practical advice

Having read so many inspiring words you may like to go to your nearest health food shop and try a few of the following remedies. You can take four to five remedies (two drops of each) at the same time in a glass of water. Rescue remedy is a good all-rounder and can be kept in the car or carried in your briefcase or handbag in case of physical shock or emotional upset.

A list of Bach flower remedies

Agrimony – For those who conceal worries behind a cheerful facade or brave face. This remedy helps positively transform worry into a genuine inner joyfulness.

Aspen – A remedy to use when feeling apprehension or vague fears for no known reason. This remedy helps a person link into higher spiritual spheres where one can find feelings of strength and confidence.

Beech – A remedy for one to use when feeling critical, intolerant or judgemental. This remedy helps one honour the different patterns of human development and behaviour.

Centaury – This remedy is for a person who is easily exploited or imposed upon; for those with weak will power. It helps one to know when to say yes.

Cerato – Use this remedy when you feel a lack of confidence in your decision making. Instead of always asking others for advice one learns to trust the inner voice.

Cherry plum – To use when experiencing uncontrolled or irrational thoughts. A very good remedy for suicidal tendencies or nervous breakdowns. Cherry plum helps one gain spiritual insight, recognise the life goal and make advances in personal development.

Chestnut bud – For those who continually repeat the same mistakes. This remedy helps one slow down, focus on the present and absorb the appropriate lesson.

Chicory – This remedy is for those with a possessive attitude, who are interfering and manipulating. This nature can be positively transformed into the eternal mother archetype who selflessly offers great love and devotion. It helps one feel secure within oneself.

Clematis – This remedy is for day-dreamers; the person who has difficulty focusing on what is going on around him/her. This helps bridge the connections between different worlds. It is useful for the writer or artist who needs to manifest creative thoughts in physical reality.

Crab apple – For the person who feels unclean, disgusted or ashamed of oneself. This remedy is known as the cleanser. It helps one see things in their proper perspective.

Elm – Use this remedy when feeling overwhelmed by responsibilities or when feeling inadequate. It enables a person to see things in their proper perspective.

Gentian – A good remedy for depressive feelings evoked by known circumstances. This remedy helps one see the light within the darkness.

Gorse – When someone says, 'Oh what's the use?', this is the correct remedy. It helps transform pessimism or defeatism into a more hopeful situation in which a person feels he/she is able to accept his/her destiny.

Heather – For a very talkative person who is overly concerned with his/her troubles and experiences. This type of person takes over a conversation always turning it to him/herself. This remedy helps a person become a more sympathetic person and a better listener.

Holly – For those who are experiencing jealousy, hatred, distrust or envy. This remedy helps one take pleasure in the achievements or successes of others. It helps one see that all is transformed through love.

Honeysuckle – A good remedy for homesickness. It is for those who are living in the past. It helps one honour the past while living in the present.

Hornbeam – For those with the 'Monday morning' feeling, weariness and a tendency to procrastinate. This remedy can help a person discover variety. It brings the feeling of being able to master the tasks that lie ahead.

Impatiens – For impatience, irritability and nervous frustration. It helps a person discover patience and empathy.

Larch – For a person who feels inferior, lacks confidence and generally expects to fail. It helps one to realise that we can only do our best.

Mimulus – For those who fear *known* things. A good remedy for those who suffer from shyness or timidity. This remedy helps one grow beyond anxieties and face the world.

Mustard – This a good remedy for depression or melancholia, especially when the feeling appears and disappears for no known reason. This remedy helps dispel gloom and despair bringing joy and light back into life.

Oak – This remedy is for the strong, reliable fighters of this world who because of illness or exhaustion suddenly feel they cannot go on. Oak helps build endurance and the ability to withstand stress.

Olive – For the times when one feels utterly exhausted. It helps one rely on inner guidance while building strength and vitality.

Pine – For feelings of guilt. It is a good remedy for those who are always apologising. Pine helps one see faults without clinging to them. It is good for self-forgiveness.

Red chestnut – This is a good remedy for those who are excessively concerned about the well-being of others. Red chestnut helps one to give positive assistance to others from a distance.

Rock rose – This a key ingredient of rescue remedy. It is useful for acute conditions of terror, fear and panic. It helps a person go beyond their fears and act in whatever way is appropriate.

Rock water – This is a very good remedy for those who are too hard on themselves, have strict views and suppress their inner needs. Rock water helps a person release unnecessary theories or principles and become more open-minded.

Scleranthus – Is for those who lack inner balance, have fluctuating moods and are indecisive.

Star of Bethlehem – Helps in dealing with shock or trauma. It is the most important ingredient of rescue remedy. It soothes and comforts pain and sorrow, giving a clear mind and inner strength.

Sweet chestnut – This is a remedy for extreme despair, especially mental despair when a person feels he has reached his limit of endurance. Sweet chestnut helps you believe in yourself again.

Vervain – Is the remedy for the overly enthusiastic or highly strung individual. It helps one use energies more wisely and with love.

Vine – For dominating, inflexible individuals who are striving for power. It helps one learn to delegate. The potential transformation is that of the wise teacher.

Walnut – For difficulty in adjusting during transition periods: (e.g. when moving, divorcing, changing occupations, retiring, etc.) It helps one resist outside influences and follow one's inner ambitions.

Water violet – Is the remedy for those who tend to withdraw from society, feel superior and, perhaps, emotionless in their isolation. It helps an individual develop a tolerant attitude and live a well-balanced life.

White chestnut – When you cannot get rid of unwanted thoughts, mental arguments and dialogues, use this remedy. It helps clear and balance the mind.

Wild oat – Helps bring peace into the decision making process about vocation and purposefulness, particularly when there is dissatisfaction because one's mission in life has not been discovered. Wild oat helps people recognise their potential and develop it. *Wild rose* – Is a good remedy for apathy, particularly when there is a lack of ambition or interest in life. Wild rose helps one find new interest in life. *Willow* – Use this remedy when life seems totally unfair or when you are feeling a victim of fate. Willow helps one find a positive attitude again. The potential transformation is the acceptance of full responsibility for one's destiny.

Rescue remedy – This is known as the first aid bottle or emergency drops. It is the most popular of the Bach flower remedies. It has saved numerous lives in emergency situations. It is made up of Star of Bethlehem (trauma), rock rose (panic), impatiens (irritability), cherry plum (fear of losing control) and clematis (for the sensation of feeling far away). The purpose of rescue remedy is to comfort, calm and reassure those who have received serious news, severe upset or startling experiences and are in shock. Rescue remedy helps to reduce the person's anguish and allows the natural healing process to begin without hindrance[5]. The idea is that under traumatic conditions our subtle bodies tend to withdraw from the physical body. Rescue remedy helps to re-integrate body-mind-spirit.

---

[1] William Shakespeare, *The Winter's Tale*, Act 4: Scene 4.

[2] Mechthild Scheffer, *Bach Flower Therapy: theory and practice* (translated from the German), Vermont: Healing Arts Press, 1988, p. 9.

[3] Reference: *Bach Flower Therapy*, p. 13

[4] Music and colour therapies are based on similar principles.

[5] Reference: *Bach Flower Therapy*, pp. 203-206

Books for further reading

Edward Bach, *The Twelve Healers and Other Remedies*(1933), *Heal Thyself* (1931) and *Step by Step* (booklets), Saffron Walden: C.W. Daniel.

Jane Evans, *Introduction to the Benefits of the Bach Flower Remedies*, Saffron Walden: C.W. Daniel, 1974.

Gurudas, *Flower Essences and Vibrational Healing*, California: Cassandra Press, 1989.

Mechthild Scheffer, *Bach Flower Therapy: theory and practice*, (translated from German), Vermont: Healing Arts Press, 1988.

Gregory Vlamis, *Flowers to the Rescue*, London: Thorsons, 1986.

Useful addresses:

Bach Flower Remedies Ltd, Mount Vernon, Sotwell, Wallingford, Oxon OX10 0PZ.

Bailey Flower Essences, 7/8 Nelson Road, Ilkley, West Yorkshire LS29 8HN.

Healing Herbs Ltd (Flower Essences), PO Box 65, Hereford HR2 0UW.

Machielle Small Wright, MAP Program for Self-healing, Perelandra Ltd, Jeffersonton VA, 22724, USA.

I ANALYSE

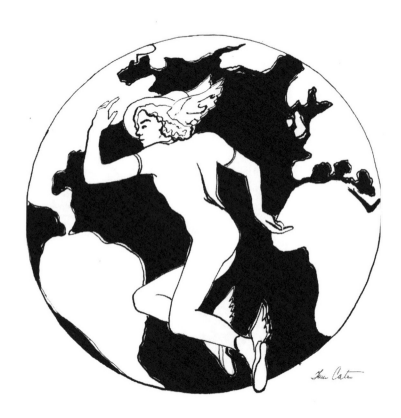

VIRGO
"Mercury, The Messenger"

VI

Homoeopathy and cell salts

*It is well to understand as early as possible in ...
life that there is just one contribution which
everyone of us can make; we can give into the
common pool of experience some comprehension
of the world as it looks to each of us.*

– Dorothea Brande

Homoeopathy

Homoeopathy[1] was developed nearly two hundred years
ago and has benefited millions of people from all walks
of life all around the globe. The word 'homoeopathy'
comes from two Greek words, homoios meaning 'same'
and pathos meaning 'suffering'. Dr Andrew Lockie
writes: 'A homeopathic remedy is one which produces the
same symptoms as those the sick person complains of,
and in doing so sharply provokes the body into throwing
them off. "Like may be cured by like", also expressed as
similia similibus curantur, is the basic principle of homeopathic therapeutics.'[2]

Controversy and proof

There is much controversy at present surrounding
homoeopathy. Lack of convincing scientific theory (to
explain how it works) is one of the great stumbling blocks
to acceptance by the general medical community. There
is no doubt that more clinical trials should be run. However, in 1854, there was an outbreak of cholera in London.
The mortality rates were compared for homoeopathic and
orthodox hospitals. The homoeopathic hospital had a
mortality rate of 16.4% while the rate at the orthodox hos-

pital was 51.8%. The Board of Health at the time attempted to suppress this information. Fortunately, Parliament demanded that the figures be recorded.

A more recent study was carried out in Glasgow in 1980 comparing homoeopathic treatment of rheumatoid arthritis with orthodox treatment by the drug aspirin. The results showed that the improvement rate was higher among the homoeopathic group, although a combination of aspirin and homoeopathic remedies was found to be the most effective treatment. However, most homoeopaths are not particularly interested in providing proof, since they know from their own experience that it works.

Homoeopathy, when used wisely, is an exceptionally safe form of medicine. Like many other alternative therapies, it relies on the body's own self-healing powers. Homoeopathy seeks to assist nature in her healing process. Allopaths (conventional doctors) treat diseases by producing a condition incompatible with or antagonistic to the condition they wish to cure or alleviate.

The father of homoeopathy

Samuel Hahnemann[3] realised that remedies and symptoms share certain key features that could interact in such a way as to banish illness. He discovered that a remedy and a disease which produce the same symptoms cancel each other out in some way. He also felt that fevers, inflammations, diarrhoea, headaches and other symptoms were not diseases, but signs that the body was attempting to return to normality. Hahnemann originally published the results of his findings in the form of a book, *Materia Medica*[4], which listed, under each remedy, the symptoms that the remedy produced in healthy people.

Homoeopaths believe that every person is different, which means that the same remedies, diets and general advice will not help everyone with the same ailment. They claim that the most effective remedy is the one that matches the physical, emotional and mental symptoms of the condition while taking into account the personality and sensitivities of the individual. It is also surprising to some people that the remedies should be taken in the least possible dose for the least possible time.

Potentisation

When a substance is diluted 1 to 100 for 12 times it is known as a 12c potency. At that potency it is unlikely that any of the original substance remains. It is difficult to explain why these infinitesimally small doses are so effective. Dr Lockie proposes that the remedy might act as a catalyst in that it speeds up the chemical working of the body and by doing so stimulates the body's innate healing powers. He also suggests that it will probably be physics, rather than chemistry, that will someday be able to explain these mysteries. The act of succussion is thought to imprint the pattern of the active substance on to the water molecules.

How to use homoeopathy

If the body's natural defence system is hampered by poor diet, negative emotions or an unhealthy environment, the remedies will be of limited benefit. Homoeopathy is not for those in search of instant solutions or easy answers; it requires careful self-monitoring. However, for serious followers, homoeopathy should lead to greater vitality and greater resistance to disease.

Dr Andrew Lockie's, *The Family Guide to Homeopathy*, is a homoeopathic first aid book written to help people decide on a sensible course of action for ailments and diseases already diagnosed. His book is readily obtainable in health food shops and book shops. It is also wise, from time to time, to see a professional homoeopath. This is particularly true in the case of cancer or other serious conditions.

At times it is necessary to use conventional surgery in conjunction with homoeopathy. However, the remedies will help the wound made by the surgeon's knife heal much more quickly. Most homoeopaths are willing to work with conventional doctors as well as involve other complementary or alternative therapies. Some homoeopaths like to use subtle methods of diagnosis such as Kirlian photography[5], iridology[6], muscle resistance testing[7] and dowsing. Homoeopaths often send patients to osteopaths, chiropractors[8] and massage therapists. The idea is to allow the body to heal itself, however, the way varies.

Obtaining remedies

There are now more than 3,000 remedies in use throughout the world, however a stock of twelve to fourteen remedies would be adequate to begin a first aid kit to have at home. Some chemists and health food shops stock a small range of remedies in the 6c potency. However, in emergencies and chronic conditions 30c remedies are the best potency to use. A full range of remedies can be bought from specialised pharmacies such as Ainsworths or Weleda[9]. Most people buy their remedies in the form of lactose (milk sugar) pilules (tablets) which have been impregnated with the named solution. To take the remedy one simply dissolves one or two tablets on the tongue (granules are better for babies and children). You must take care not to touch the tablets since this can lessen the effectiveness of the remedy. Ointments, creams, lotions and mother tinctures[10] can also be used. Store your remedies in a cool, dark, dry place. If your child eats your collection, don't worry: they aren't poisonous and they won't harm her, but she may experience diarrhoea from the lactose sugar.

Taking remedies

It is best to take remedies twenty minutes before or after eating or drinking. It is also wise to avoid strongly flavoured foods, herbs and spices such as mint, garlic, coffee, curries and tobacco, as well as perfume and most essential oils.

In acute[11] situations, doses can be taken up to every half an hour until symptoms are relieved or up to a maximum of ten doses. Dr Lockie stresses that there is absolutely no point in continuing to take a remedy once the symptoms have started to disappear.

In chronic[12] conditions, 6c remedies are usually taken three times a day for up to fourteen days and 30c remedies every twelve hours for a few days – the stronger the mental and emotional symptoms, the higher the potency; the stronger the physical symptoms, the lower the potency. Remember that you want the smallest dose for the least possible time. Once the body has received the message, the innate healing systems will do the rest.

If the symptoms get neither better nor worse, you have probably selected the wrong remedy. Homoeopathic remedies usually can be taken with orthodox drugs, although many drugs block the effect of the remedies. Do not stop taking any drugs without consulting your doctor first. If in doubt, or if you are pregnant, contact a professional. The remedies listed below are to be considered an introduction to homoeopathy and its properties; it should not be used to select remedies. If you are interested in obtaining and using these remedies, please refer to Dr Lockie's book or consult a qualified homoeopath.

Starter remedies

Aconite 30c – from the plant also known as monkshood.
• Mental symptoms alleviated: Many aspects of behaviour dictated by fear.
• Physical symptoms alleviated: Fever which comes on suddenly, with skin hot, dry and angry-looking.

Apis 30c – from whole honey bees dissolved in alcohol.
• Mental symptoms alleviated: Depression and irritability.
• Physical symptoms alleviated: Watery swellings on mouth or eyelids; swelling which spreads to throat and hinders breathing; oedema[13]; scanty urination. (Increased urination indicates that Apis is working well.)

Arnica 30c – from the plant Arnica montana or leopard's bane, found particularly in the Swiss Alps.
• Mental symptoms alleviated: Hopelessness; indifference; shock.
• Physical symptoms alleviated: Bruises; sore muscles; sprained joints; sore gums after dentistry; black eyes.

Belladonna 30c – from the plant Atropa belladonna or the deadly nightshade.
• Mental symptoms alleviated: Restlessness; racing imagination; hallucinations.
• Physical symptoms alleviated: Fever which comes on suddenly, individual has hot, flushed skin, pounding pulse, staring eyes, and becomes delirious. Also good for earache and throbbing headaches.

Cantharis 30c – derived from a species of beetle misleadingly called the Spanish fly. A first resort for people who look as if they are suffering intensely.
• Mental symptoms alleviated: Rage; anxiety; screaming; violence.
• Physical symptoms alleviated: Cystitis with scalding inflammation that worsens rapidly and cannot be

ignored; also diarrhoea that burns and scalds.

Carbo veg 30c – from vegetable charcoal, made from beech, birch or poplar wood. Its main action is removal of mucus from the digestive system.
• Mental symptoms alleviated: Lack of mental energy.
• Physical symptoms alleviated: Digestive problems, no matter what kinds of food are eaten; wind; heartburn; sour belching.

Chamomilla 6c – from German chamomile. Individuals who respond best to this remedy have a very low pain threshold and are often bad-tempered and complaining. Complaints often begin with the words, 'I can't bear ...'
• Mental symptoms alleviated: Inner turmoil; bad-temper.
• Physical symptoms alleviated: Moaning and crying in sleep; tearing pains in general; in women, heavy periods accompanied by severe labour-like pains.

Euphrasia 6c – from Euphrasia officinalis, common eye-bright. This remedy is traditionally used as a cure for eye ailments.
• Physical symptoms alleviated: Watering eyes; conjunctivitis[14].

Hypericum 6c and 30c – from Hypericum perforatum, St John's wort. It is mainly used to treat nerve injuries.
• Mental symptoms alleviated: Drowsiness; depression.
• Physical symptoms alleviated: Concussion; neuralgia[15].

Ledum 6c – from the plant Ledum palustre, also known as wild rosemary. This remedy is traditionally used to heal puncture wounds and soothe pains which ascend from the lower part of the body.
• Mental symptoms alleviated: Wanting to be left alone; impatience; working oneself into a state of anger.
• Physical symptoms alleviated: Stiff joints that loosen up when bathed in cold water.

Nux vomica – from the seeds of the plant also known as poison nut tree.
• Mental symptoms alleviated: Fanatical precision and tidiness; irritability.
• Physical symptoms alleviated: Hangovers from too much alcohol; indigestion and vomiting; 24-hour flu, with shivering and stiff, aching muscles.

Pulsatilla 6c – from the leaves of the plant also known as Anemone pratensis, the wind flower.
• Mental symptoms alleviated: Depression; longing for attention and affection.
• Physical symptoms alleviated: Blocked up nose at night, runny nose during day.

Rhus toxicodendron 6c – from the leaves of the plant also known as poison oak and closely related to poison ivy.
• Mental symptoms alleviated: Bursting into tears for no particular reason; depression or thoughts of suicide; fear of being poisoned.
• Physical symptoms alleviated: Eczema; stiff, painful muscles which seize up with rest but loosen up with exercise or heat; stiffness in lower back.

Ruta 6c – From Ruta graveolens, rue, also known as herb-of-grace and herb-of-repentance. Herbals refer to rue as 'an antidote to all dangerous poisons' and as a defence against witches! In homoeopathy ruta has virtue against restlessness and bruising.
• Mental symptoms alleviated: Dissatisfaction with self and others.
• Physical symptoms alleviated: Tendon injuries and bruised bones; sciatica, often worse at night when lying down; deep aching in the bones; painful bruises.

Cell salts

Cell salts (also called tissue salts) occupy a unique place in homoeopathy. Most homoeopathic remedies are obtained from plant or animal material and are not typical constituents of the body. Cell salts, however, are found naturally as components of the physical body and, what is more, they do not usually conform with the homoeopathic 'like cures like' idea. That is, cell salts, do not usually produce the illness in a healthy person that they would cure in a sick individual. Their action seems to be more that of a catalyst. They act as a stimulant in bringing about a cure. Some say they provide 'information' to the body to better utilise its mineral constituents. In any case, what is certain is that in their potentised form, cell salts can be highly effective remedies for a wide range of conditions.

Samuel Hahnemann, the father of modern homoeopathy, was the first scientific healer to investigate cell salts as therapeutic agents. He worked with salt, silica, lime and potash as substances having potential medicinal force.

Following Hahnemann's lead, a German doctor, by the name of W.H. Schussler, working in the 1870s, studied the inorganic constituents of cremated human remains. Schussler found that twelve simple minerals were the most abundant components of cremated remains. He deduced that these minerals were essential to our physiological processes and that a deficiency of any of them would result in disharmony to the entire organism. While Schussler's theory seems a bit simplistic in the light of today's more thorough analysis of the body's constituents, his discovery nonetheless gives alternative healing some very valuable remedies. Schussler himself, maintained that these remedies had a physiological –chemical effect on the body and did not act homoeopathically. Yet these remedies take on considerable value after homoeopathic potentisation.

In preparing cell salts, the original mineral is mixed with milk sugar in a ratio of one part mineral to nine parts milk sugar. These are crushed, ground and pulverised together for at least one hour. The result is a 1x potentisation which experience has shown is not very useful. So one part of this 1x mixture is blended with another nine parts of milk sugar, pulverised again for an hour for a 2x potency. Since the 2x is not particularly valuable, it is then mixed with one part to another nine parts of milk sugar, pulverised again for an hour to produce the very useful 3x potency. Thus we arrive at a substance that contains one thousandth of the original substance. And it is in this proportion that it begins to be truly effective!

The described dilution and grinding (trituration) is continued further producing another stage, 6x, which experience has shown to be extremely valuable. (This is one millionth of the original mineral!) Why the intervening potencies such as 4x or 5x are of lesser value no one can say. The next useful potency after 6x is 12x. After the 12x, the 30x is found to be of value.

Some formats for preparing cell salts offer an even greater dilution. Instead of mixing one part mineral with nine parts milk sugar, the blend will be one part mineral with one hundred parts milk sugar. The grinding procedure described above produces a 1C potency. One part of this is mixed with another one hundred parts of milk sugar for the 2C potency, and so on. Whether to use the x potency or the C potency seems, at this time, to be a subjective choice.

How do cell salts work?

Keeping in mind the basic belief behind most alternative therapies (that the body is constantly self-repairing and self-renewing), then the cell salts must provide either information to properly guide the self-repair or provide some essential physical ingredient. Many healers believe that cell salts provide both. Thus they see cell salts as a kind of bridge remedy. That is, in its lower potencies it effects the physical body while in the higher potencies it directs the mental or ethereal aspects.

The following outline provides a very simplified guide to cell salts. Please read more about them or consult a practitioner in the field before using cell salts. Although they are generally very safe, some people have reported side-effects. Like all medicines, cell salts must be used wisely.

PRIMARY FUNCTIONS:

Phosphates: Calc Phos – bones and teeth
Ferr Phos – exhaustion, inflammation
Kali Phos – nervousness, anxiety
Nat Phos – too much sugar or fat
Mag Phos – cramps, bloating, asthma

Chlorides: Kali Mur – catarrh, rheumatic pain
Nat Mur – too much salt

Sulphates: Calc Sulph – unhealthy discharges
Nat Sulph – eliminating toxic fluids
Kali Sulph – common cold, skin conditions

Others: Calc Fluor – rebuild elastic fibres of muscles
Silicea – cleanser/conditioner and eliminator

1 Also spelt 'homeopathy'.

2 Dr Andrew Lockie, *The Family Guide to Homeopathy: the safe form of medicine for the future*, London: Hamish Hamilton, 1990, p. 9.

3 'The father of homoeopathy', was born in Dresden, Germany in 1755.

4 A modern *Materia Medica* can easily be obtained from Ainsworths, a homoeopathic pharmacy in London. See list of addresses at end of chapter.

5 See Section IV: Energy therapies.

6 Iridology is an ancient diagnostic technique through analysis of the iris of the eye.

7 Basically the strength of a person is tested while holding a remedy or food. If the patient is strong then the substance will strenghten them, if weak (as is usually the case with sugar) the substance should be avoided.

8 Osteopaths and chiropractors manipulate the spine.

9 See useful addresses.

10 Mother tinctures should be diluted: usually 10 drops of mother tincture to 0.25 litre (half pint) of boiled and cooled water. Some remedies are for external use, others are for internal use. Make sure to read the label or if ordering, be sure to clearly explain what you need.

11 Characterised by sharpness or severity.

12 Marked by long duration, by frequent recurrence over a long time, and often by slowly progressing seriousness.

13 Abnormal accumulation of fluids in body tissues, showing as puffiness under the skin, especially around the ankles. Many women, especially before menstruation, in hot weather, or as a result of prolonged standing, develop a minor form of oedema. Self-help: cut down on salt and try to lose weight.

14 Inflammation of the conjunctiva, the transparent covering of the eye, due to infection or allergy.

15 Damaged or inflamed nerves.

Books for further reading

W. Boericke, *Materia Medica with Repertory*, Philadelphia: Boericke and Tafel, 1927.

J.B. Chapman and Edward L. Perry, *The Biochemic Handbook* (revised), St. Louis: Formur,1976.

Dr Ann Clover, *Homoeopathic First Aid: 20 useful medicines for day-to-day problems*, London: Thorsons Publishers Limited, 1990.

Dr Peter Gilbert, *Thorsons Complete Guide to Homoeopathically Prepared Mineral Tissue Salts*, London: Thorsons Publishers Limited, 1989.

Dr Andrew Lockie, *The Family Guide to Homeopathy: the safe form of medicine for the future*, London: Hamish Hamilton, 1989.

Dr Andrew Lockie and Dr Nicola Geddes, *The Woman's Guide to Homeopathy: the natural way to a healthier life for women*, London: Hamish Hamilton, 1992.

Dr S.R. Phatak, *Phatak's Materia Medica of Homoeopathic Medicines*, London: Foxlee-Vaughan Publishers, 1988.

George Vithoulkas, *Homoeopathy: medicine of the new man*, London: Thorsons Publishers Limited, 1979.

Useful addresses

The British Homoeopathic Association, 27a Devonshire Street, London WC1N 1RJ.

Ainsworth (homoeopathic pharmacy), 38 New Cavendish Street, London W1M 7LH.

Weleda (UK) Ltd (licensed manufacturer), Heanor Road, Ilkeston, Derbyshire DE7 8DR.

WE BALANCE

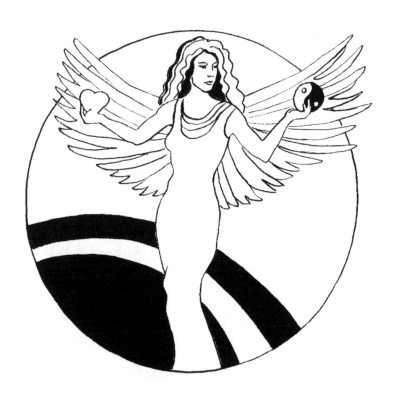

LIBRA
"Balancing the I Ching and the Heart"

VII

Nutritional medicine

Let food be your medicine, and medicine your food.
— Hippocrates

The range of nutritional advice is vast. Many arguments are fought over the so-called ideal diet. Should we eat meat? Should we have butter or margarine? Is the macrobiotic diet best? The list is endless. Many conditions have been linked with the overconsumption of refined carbohydrates and animal fats including obesity, degenerative diseases, dental decay, coronary artery disease, diabetes, gallstones and diverticular diseases. Undernutrition is prevalent in poorer countries, but malnutrition can occur anywhere as a result of poor food choice and a dependence on a large amount of heavily refined foods. To avoid the diseases of overconsumption, the World Health Organisation has redefined the ideal diet to conform more closely to that of our hunter–gatherer forefathers.

There are four main categories of diet: a western omnivore diet includes refined and processed foods; an omnivore wholefood diet includes all types of wholefoods (foods not processed, treated or refined by industry); a vegan diet includes no animal protein of any kind; and a lacto–vegetarian diet includes milk products and, sometimes, eggs as the only sources of animal protein. None of these diets is the correct one. It varies from individual to individual. Every person has different needs. Listed below are a few nutritional guidelines, but the rest must come from your own research and intuition.

Nutritional guidelines

1. Eat foods that are as near as possible to their natural state. That is, avoid tins, packets and additives.

2. Food should be as organic or as free from toxins or harmful additives as possible.

3. At least half of an adult's diet should be made up of raw or lightly cooked vegetables and fruit. Children, the infirm and the elderly may have difficulty digesting raw foods, but home-made vegetable soups can provide many essential nutrients.

4. Avoid saturated fats (fats from animal sources) since they contribute to heart disease. Animals raised for meat are often deprived of exercise, sunshine and fresh air. They are also fed chemicals, residues of which can end up in your body. So, if you eat meat, then try to find free-range products. Eat free-range eggs, since they are free of antibiotic residues and other chemicals that are added to the feed of battery hens in an attempt to keep the poor things 'healthy'. Also, according to some reports, battery eggs have twice as much saturated fat as free-range eggs.

5. Food additives place an enormous burden on the liver and kidneys. People suffering from allergies, arthritis, kidney stones and urinary tract infections should avoid them completely.

6. As we all know, sugar causes tooth decay and excess weight gain. Excess sugar consumption is also associated with artery disease leading to heart attacks. It can cause imbalances in the body's blood sugar maintenance and can lead to diabetes. Honey, in small quantities, is a healthier alternative to sugar. It is digested much more easily and is not as damaging to the teeth. Maple syrup, molasses and raw sugar are other healthier alternatives.

7. Excess alcohol can cause the same metabolic imbalances as sugar and it eventually leads to liver damage. Alcohol should be avoided totally during pregnancy. Some studies have shown that one or two glass of organic wine a day may be beneficial to the cardiovascular system. This is a personal decision.

8. Caffeine is an addictive stimulant which can damage the kidneys and deplete the body's calcium levels. Studies have found a link between caffeine intake and anxiety. If you cannot give up caffeine, do limit yourself to one and not more than three small cups a day. Some studies have shown that organic filtered coffee (if taken black) contains minerals that are beneficial to the body. Remember, we all have different needs.

Use this list as a quick reference to improve your diet over a period of time. This does not take allergies or other illnesses into account. You must listen to your body. Write this list on a piece of colourful paper and attach it to your refrigerator.

Basic awareness guidelines

1. Buy organically grown food when you can.

2. Add brown rice, oats, beans, lentils and nuts to your diet.

3. Eat lots of fresh fruit and vegetables.

4. Use cold-pressed oils (for instance, virgin olive oil) instead of butter.

5. Cut down on all fats, especially butter, cream and full-fat cheeses.

6. Sweeten your food sparingly.

7. Restrict your salt intake. Use herbs for flavouring instead.

8. When eating meat, select white over red meats. Try to buy organic or free-range meats if possible.

9. Try soya milk and tofu. If you must have dairy products, use low fat products and keep milk consumption down to half pint per day.

10. Avoid processed foods and chemical additives.

11. Cook your food with love. Take time out to enjoy your meal. Make the table look nice. Light a candle. Put on some classical music. Eat slowly. Enjoy!

12. Know that the food you are eating is nourishing your body in the best possible way.

Write out your normal diet over the course of a typical one-week period. Look over the guidelines again and think about the ways in which your diet could be improved. Many large supermarkets now carry organic produce. Are you familiar with your local health food shop? Write out a list of new foods that you would like to introduce into your diet. Be daring. Be creative!

There are many diets. One that has recently had a lot of attention because of some rather spectacular results is macrobiotics. I am not stating that this is the best diet, only that it is an option. It gives you a starting point for future discoveries into your own health and your own needs.

Introduction to macrobiotics

Being the source of life, food is the primary cause of, and our basic tool for treating any type of imbalance.
– Michio Kushi

Macrobiotics evolved from the 4000 year old traditions of Oriental medicine. Macrobiotics is not just a diet, it is a way of living. The basic tools of macrobiotics include a wholesome, natural diet, self-reflection, self-diagnosis skills and simple home care remedies. The macrobiotic diet is said to calm the mind and emotions, while renewing the body.

Supportive research at Harvard Medical School indicates that a macrobiotic diet may be one of the best ways to prevent heart disease, since it lowers levels of cholesterol and the blood pressure[1]. In Boston, where the Kushi Institute for macrobiotic studies is located, so many individuals have switched to the macrobiotic diet that both McDonalds and Howard Johnson's are now offering a macrobiotic breakfast. Recent scientific research into the macrobiotic diet has brought impressive results. Studies have shown that a macrobiotic diet can help with the following conditions: allergies, candida yeast infections, diabetes, digestive disorders, heart disease, premenstrual symptoms, anaemia, hyperactivity in children and many types of cancer. Macrobiotics is also noted for its ability to slow down or arrest the development of AIDS. At the United Nations, a Macrobiotic Society with 150 members was started by Katsuhide Katatani, UN Development Director for Southeast Asia, who healed his stomach cancer on a macrobiotic diet.

Macrobiotics is about balance and harmony, the creation of health and happiness, and the freedom to choose our own direction of life. It is based on an understanding of the ancient concept of yin and yang. This concept allows a vision of unity to develop in all aspects of life. A mind bod, spirit connection develops as well as a connection between food, our physical health, moods, emotions, behaviour and thinking.

Yin is the name given to the energy of movement that is expanding or outward-moving. Yang is the name given to the energy of movement that is contracting or inward-moving. For example, trees are created by the yin tendency since their leaves expand upwards and outwards. Animals are created by a more concentrated or yang tendency. By looking at the yin and yang qualities of plants, foods or individuals, we can learn how to achieve balance and health in the body and in life. Heat is produced by contraction and so is considered yang, while coolness is produced by expansion and therefore considered yin. There are also two basic aspects to our thinking which are controlled by the two hemispheres of our brain. The left side is associated with a more contractive or yang nature which includes analytical, logical and rational thought. The right side is associated with more yin work such as intuitive thinking used in creative and healing activities. Instead of being frustrated by ambiguity, Kushi describes these variations as being part of the paradoxical nature of reality. Nothing is right or wrong, yin or yang, there are only tendencies.

In the growth of plants a root growing downwards is compact, hard and is associated with the yang force. A leafy plant growing upwards is formed more by the use of rising yin energy. All these pairs are both opposite and complementary, since plants and animals depend on each other for survival. Plants take in carbon dioxide and give out oxygen during photosynthesis, while animals take in oxygen and give out carbon dioxide.

In nature there are many alternations of yin and yang, such as the seasons, the daily cycles of night and day, the lunar cycle and the tides. In the human being there are also cycles between emotions, and between life and death. The chart below illustrates some examples of yin and yang.

	YIN	**YANG**
Life form:	plants	animals
Activity:	less active	more active
Colour[2]:	violet – blue – green – yellow – orange – red	
Direction:	upwards	downwards
Weight:	lighter	heavier
Light:	darker	brighter
Texture:	softer	harder
Sex:	female	male
Attitude:	gentle, receptive	active, outgoing
Dimension:	space	time

Taking the principles of yin and yang into the diet, we see that animal foods like meat, poultry, eggs and fish are more yang than plant foods like grains, vegetables, seeds, nuts and fruit. Another principle is that plant extracts or plant derivatives are usually more yin than the plants they are taken from, such as sugar, syrups, fruit juices, alcohol, tea, coffee, most drugs and medications. This divides foods into three categories: yang animal foods, yin plant extracts, and plant foods that fall in between. Some foods do not fit so neatly into these categories, e.g. dairy foods such as milk, yoghurt and cream which fall into the yin category. Also, salt, which has a strong contractive quality, is therefore yang. When we eat a yang food we are automatically attracted to eating a yin food to make up the balance, and vice versa. When you consume alcohol (yin), you are probably tempted to eat salty snacks (yang). If you carefully observe the foods you are eating, you will also be able to tune into the foods you need to find harmony and balance.

FOODS

More Yang	More Balanced	More Yin
salt	grains	sugar
meat	beans	honey
eggs	vegetables	molasses
poultry	seeds	tea
fish	nuts	coffee
seafood	fruit	alcohol
hard salty cheese		spices
		herbs
		fruit juices
		yoghurt
		milk

A main macrobiotic principle of eating is that the majority of foods in your diet should be chosen from the central, balanced category. Being the source of life, balanced food creates a balanced individual. Eating a combination of both extreme yin and yang foods causes a variety of physical problems including arteriosclerosis[3], arthritis, breast cysts and cancer, lung cancer, kidney stones, cataracts and pneumonia. It can also cause emotional disturbances such as paranoia. Physical problems caused by an extreme yang diet include: hepatitis, appendicitis, jaundice, gout, liver cancer, headaches at the back of the head. Physical problems from an excessively yin diet include: asthma, leukaemia, cystitis, varicose veins, pleurisy, hernia, colitis, meningitis, stomach ulcers and headaches at the front of the head. It can also cause nervousness, anxiety, over-emotional behaviour and can eventually lead to such problems as schizophrenia.

By following the macrobiotic idea of eating a centrally balanced diet, it is possible to avoid all of these illnesses. There are also other benefits such as increased level of vitality and energy, deeper and more restful sleep, natural level of body weight, increased flexibility of the body and greater stamina. Health problems that cause minor inconveniences such as poor circulation, coughs and colds, blocked sinuses, headaches and sore throats, gradually disappear.

When we eat a balanced diet, our hormonal and nervous systems gradually become balanced. Deep tension is transformed into inner calm, worry into confidence, depression into joy, impatience into patience and irritability into a good sense of humour. As you achieve unity in yourself, unity can also be achieved between physical and material aspects of life.

When designing a balanced diet, a macrobiotic practitioner would select foods from the central, balanced scale including grains, beans and vegetables, small amounts of fish, fruit, seeds, nuts and some other foods. Children are growing at a rapid rate and need milk, sugars, calcium and other minerals. After the second year of life, dairy products will begin forming fat deposits in arteries. Milk is not necessary as a source of calcium since calcium can also be obtained in greens such as kale, parsley and watercress, as well as from nuts such as almonds and hazelnuts, and beans like chickpeas and soya beans. Dairy products are also mucus-forming and are a primary cause of mucus in the lungs, sinuses and ears. An ideal macrobiotic diet for an adult excludes all dairy products including goat's milk.

Michio Kushi has designed a diet plan suited for people living in Great Britain, North America and Northern Europe. Half of the diet is made up of whole cereal grains including: brown rice, barley, wheat, buckwheat and corn (maize) as well as various flours made from whole grains like wholemeal bread, noodles and porridge oats. A third of the diet is made up of a wide range of vegetables. Sea vegetables form 3–4% of the diet and play a vital role due to their high mineral and vitamin content.

The rest is made up of 5% soup, 5–10% beans and 5% seeds, nuts, fish, seasonings and condiments.

A typical summer menu

BREAKFAST
Rolled oat porridge
Boiled brocoli

LUNCH
Fried rice with onion, mushrooms,
beansprouts, and spring onions
Sauerkraut

SUPPER
Miso soup
Pressure-cooked short-grain rice
Carrots & kombu[4]
Cucumber & wakame[5] salad with rice vinegar
Strawberry jelly[6]

A typical winter menu

BREAKFAST
Soft millet cooked with onion and mushroom

LUNCH
Rice & chestnuts
Steamed brocoli

SUPPER
Aduki bean soup
Pressure-cooked short-grain rice and barley
Sauté of carrot, swede and Brussels sprouts
Boiled leeks mixed with umeboshi plum dressing

Miso is a dark paste made by fermenting soya beans with sea salt, and often a grain like barley, wheat or rice. Miso is particularly good to use on a regular basis. It provides vitamin B12, and is a good source of easily digested protein. Unpasteurised miso provides live enzymes that aid digestion and promote bowel health. A small quantity added to any soup gives a rich and full flavour.

Try making your own miso soup:

Vegetable miso soup

Half cup onions thinly sliced.
3–4 inch (8–10 cm) piece of wakame seaweed
1 pint (550 ml) water
half to one tablespoon miso

Variations: cauliflower and onion; wakame and daikon (mooli); corn cut from a cob and Chinese cabbage.

Quickly rinse the wakame in water to remove excess salt and soak in half cup water for 5 minutes, then slice into half-inch (1 cm) pieces. Place the wakame with its soaking water and onions in a saucepan and add the rest of the water. Bring to the boil, cover and simmer for 10–15 minutes or until tender. Reduce flame[7] to very low so there is no bubbling. Puree the miso with a quarter cup of the soup and return to the soup. Allow to cook for 3 to 4 minutes without bubbling to preserve the beneficial enzymes in the miso, and serve. Garnish with chopped parsley, spring onion, watercress or grated root ginger.

The soup should not taste too salty nor too bland. A little more miso will be needed in the winter and a little less in the summer. Barley miso is the most balanced and the best to use regularly. For variations add the extra vegetables listed above.

[1] See *Diet for a Strong Heart* by Micho Kushi.

[2] Violet is the most yin colour. Green and yellow are more neutral colours. Red is the most yang.

[3] Slow clogging up and hardening of arteries due to build-up of fatty deposits on smooth inner walls which disrupts blood flow and eventually leads to weakened artery walls. This is a serious condition when vital organs are effected.

[4] Kombu is a sea vegetable used to soften beans and make them more digestible.

[5] Wakame is known as 'the women's seaweed'. It is beneficial for the reproductive organs and to help regulate women's cycles. It is traditionally used in Oriental medicine to purify the blood, strengthen the intestines, skin and hair.

[6] This is made with a natural gelatine called agar-agar.

[7] Macrobiotic practitioners prefer cooking over a flame on a gas cooker. They argue that electric stoves and microwaves kill the vital force contained within the food.

Useful books

Oliver Cowmeadow, *Introduction to Macrobiotics*, London: Thorsons Publishing Limited, 1987.

Michio Kushi and Philip Jannetta, *Macrobiotics and Oriental Medicine*, Tokyo and New York: Japan Publications, 1991.

Michio Kushi and Martha C. Cotterel with Mark N. Mead, *AIDS, Macrobiotics, and Natural Immunity*, Tokyo and New York: Japan Publications, 1990.

Aveline Kushi, *Aveline Kushi's Complete Guide to Macrobiotic Cooking*, New York: Warner Books, 1985.

Kristina Turner, *The Self-Healing Cookbook*, Washington: Earthtones Press, 1989.

Useful address:

The Kushi Institute, 188 Old Street, London EC1V 9BP.

I CREATE

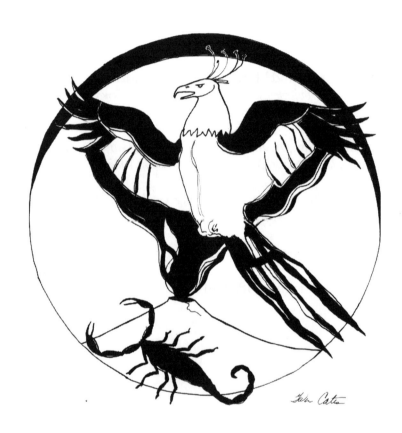

SCORPIO
"Scorpio Rising"

VIII

Reflexology

If one persists,
there comes a time
when one is victorious.
Victory is to the persistent.
– The Mother

Reflexology is a form of foot massage. Massage can relax a patient, bring emotional relief and improve the circulation. However, reflexologists take this theory further, maintaining that there is an interrelationship between certain parts of the body and points on the feet. Reflexology is based on Eastern philosophies. Those that follow Chinese Taoism say that humankind should strive as far as possible to be at one with nature. Reflexologists feel that this type of treatment is one of the ways that the relationship between the universe and humankind can be demonstrated.

Western scientists do not easily accept these theories, and there is as yet no scientific evidence that proves the effectiveness of reflexology. However, as is the case with many alternative therapies, we must rely on case histories and our own personal experiences for proof. This is not necessarily a negative aspect since it teaches us to rely on our own judgement and to look for our own intuitive and innate wisdom for our understanding of the world.

Throughout recorded history, Europeans, Asians and Americans have intuitively discovered various points where they could apply pressure and bring relief from pain. In India and China, there are 5,000 year old records of treatment by pressure points on the feet. The link between points on the feet and internal organs of the body was discovered and is still used in the treatment of disease by North American Indians. It appears that the technique died out during the Middle Ages and then re-emerged in the 16th Century.

The birth of modern reflexology took place at the turn of the century. Dr William FitzGerald (1872–1942), an American ear, nose and throat specialist, is recognised as the founder of zone therapy. Dr FitzGerald and Dr Edwin F. Bowers combined their knowledge and skills to produce a book which contains practical therapeutic proposals and recommendations for zone therapy. Dr FitzGerald went on to run courses and produce diagrams of the zones of the feet and the corresponding ten zones of the body. He is responsible for turning reflexology into a science.

An American masseuse, Eunice Ingham, who was trained in zone therapy, developed a pressure massage for the feet. It is known as the Ingham method of compression massage and is considered the cornerstone of modern reflexology.

A reflexologist will tell you that a person's feet clearly reflect what the body wants to say. When a reflexologist reads the feet she[1] looks for discoloration, patches of pigmentation and cracks in the skin of heels and toes, and ascertains the amount of tension in the patient and the temperature and smell of the feet. Each indicates an imbalance of some sort. It is then her job to interpret these signs.

A reflexologist divides the body into ten vertical grid zones, which correspond to the ten grid zones of the feet (dividing the feet from heel to toe into ten fields). These vertical zones allow the therapist to locate the organs of the body in their longitudinal relationship to one another. She then divides the body into three transverse (or horizontal) zones which are related to the skeleton. The head and neck are represented in zone I, the thorax (chest) and upper abdomen in zone II, and the abdomen and pelvic region in zone III. This is again seen in the feet since the toes relate to the head and neck, the middle of the foot relates to the thorax and upper abdomen, while the abdomen and pelvis are related to the base of the foot or heel.

Generally speaking, every organ has a corresponding reflex zone in the feet, lying in the same zone in the feet as in the body. Thus you find the organs of the right half of the body in the right foot and the organs of the left side of the body in the left foot. Organs that are paired in the body are found in their corresponding zones on both feet. Single organs are found only once, in either the left or right foot, and conform to their anatomical position. Organs that lie in the centre of the body are found in both feet.

In general, the reflex zones of the organs can be pressed or palpated on the plantar aspect (bottom or sole) of the foot, whilst those associated with bones, muscles and nerves lie on the dorsal aspect (top of the foot).

Reflexology offers many benefits. It is said to induce a state of relaxation and can bring emotional relief. It improves the circulation, increases the dynamic force throughout the body and improves the general condition of the body.

There are several contraindications to (or reasons to avoid) reflexology. They include: heart problems[2], cancer[3], pregnancy[4], deep vein thrombosis[5] and people who have recently undergone surgery[6]. When treating other people you should always avoid direct pressure on calluses, corns, injuries and wounds. Never treat anyone suffering from a contagious illness. If you suffer from any of the listed conditions, or are in doubt, do not try the practical self-reflexology exercise until you speak to a professional.

Self-reflexology exercise

It is difficult to give yourself a whole self-reflexology massage treatment. However, it is possible to treat some reflexes on your feet, especially if you know which ones are out of balance.

Sit down and make yourself as comfortable as possible. Remember that the points on the right and left feet vary, so make sure you have the correct foot. One advantage with self-reflexology is that your feet are always with you. Keep in mind that weak stimuli are beneficial, strong stimuli are detrimental and very strong stimuli are harmful.

Look at the diagram provided at the end of the chapter and locate the area of the solar plexus. Using the balls of the thumbs, press this area gently but firmly three times. Press the reflex in as you breathe in, relax the pressure as you breathe out. Most reflexology treatments begin and end with this treatment since it has a great influence on the autonomic nervous system[7].

Next, find the position of the pituitary reflex located on the middle of the large toe. The pituitary gland is known as the master gland since it influences almost all the other glands of the endocrine system. Press the pituitary reflex gently three times. Feel yourself coming back into harmony and balance.

The reflexes of the neck muscles are located at the base of the big toe. Tension in the neck muscles can cause neck pain. Rub around the base of the big toe and then, rotate the toe in a clockwise and then a counter-clockwise direction. It is possible to relax the neck muscles to some extent by carefully rotating the big toe.

Find the lung reflex on the ball of the sole and press gently. Then find any other area that you know is currently affecting your state of health and treat that reflex point. Do not be surprised if you feel some tenderness in that area. Remember to repeat the sequence on the other foot.

Once you have mastered the sequence on your own feet you may want to try treating a friend. These are only a few of the reflex points. You may want to gradually increase your knowledge and awareness by taking a class or finding a more in depth reflexology chart.

---

[1] I have used the feminine form since the majority of relexologists are female.

[2] People with pacemakers should avoid reflexology treatment.

[3] A reflexology treatment could cause cancer to spread. However, in a case of terminal cancer, that may not matter and the person may benefit more from therapeutic touch. We remind you to take responsibility for your choices.

[4] A reflexology treatment could cause miscarriage in a weak pregnancy. The best rule is to avoid treatment during pregnancy if you are new to the technique.

[5] Deep vein thrombosis is defined as the presence of a blood clot in a deep vein, usually in a leg or the lower abdomen, which obstructs the return of blood to the heart; pressure in veins and capillaries below the clot rises, causing pain, swelling, and sometimes dark red discolouration of the skin. Reflexology should be avoided in this case since it could cause the clot to move.

[6] Avoid reflexology for 3 months after minor surgery and 6 months after major surgery.

[7] This is the division of the nervous system that supplies all body structures over which we have no voluntary control.

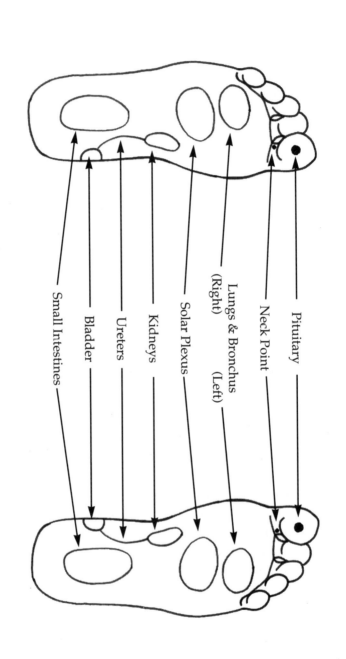

Small Intestines

Bladder

Ureters

Kidneys

Solar Plexus

Lungs & Bronchus
(Right)   (Left)

Neck Point

Pituitary

Useful books

Hanne Marquardt, *Reflex Zone Therapy of the Feet: a textbook for therapists*, London: Thorsons, 1983.

Astrid I. Goosmann-Legger, *Zone Therapy Using Foot Massage*, Saffron Walden: C.W. Daniel, 1983.

Chris Stormer, *Reflexology*, London: Headway, 1992.

Pauline Wills, *The Reflexology and Colour Therapy Workbook*, Shaftesbury: Element, 1992.

Useful addresses

Association of Reflexologists, 37 Standale Grove, Ruislip, Middlesex HA4 7UA.

British Reflexology Association, 12 Pond Road, London SE3 9JL.

International Institute of Reflexology, 28 Holyfield Avenue, Friern Barnet, London N11 3BY.

College of Reflexology, 9 Mead Road, Shenley, Radlett, Herts WD7 9DA.

I PERCEIVE

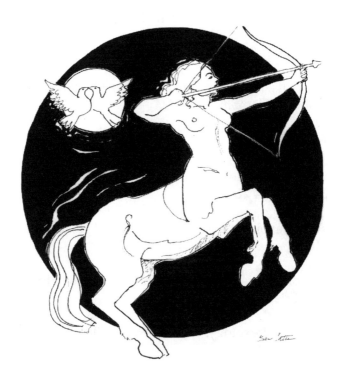

SAGITTARIUS
"Centaur Archer"

IX

Sound therapy

The entire universe is like a lyre tuned by some excellent artificer, whose strings are separate species of the universal whole. Anyone who knew how to touch these dextrously and make them vibrate would draw forth marvellous harmonies. In himself, man is wholly analogous to the universal lyre.
– John Dee

Sound is one of the oldest methods of healing. Ancient ideas run through Greek, Chinese, Persian, Indian, Native American and primitive peoples. There was song and dance in most of the old healing rituals. Ancient Chinese healers used singing stones made of thin, flat plates of jade. When the stones were struck they gave off musical tones. 'Amen' comes from the more ancient 'Aum' or 'OM' which is associated with the God-force.

Laurel Elizabeth Keyes' book *Toning: the Creative Power of the Voice,* is considered a classic by many sound therapists. She has also done experiments on cancer cells, concentrating on tuning the body as a whole. Her work is well respected. Keyes believes that the creative force is enslaved and directed by the mind. When the mind and feelings are in conflict, the feelings usually win. The wall of separation lying between the subconscious and conscious mind causes a great deal of trouble and sorrow. Keyes has found that toning forms a bridge between the conscious and subconscious. This allows holistic healing to take place.

The Greek philosopher and mathematician, Pythagoras (530 B.C.), saw the whole universe as a harmony of the spheres and taught that sound was a creative force. He also believed that music held therapeutic benefits for the body. Today, sound therapists feel that our actions and reactions result from sound. We use words to create our realities.

Toning

It is important to maintain a feeling of enthusiasm in your life. When you pour love and interest into what you are doing, you are supporting and influencing that reality in a positive way. Toning or even verbal prayer helps the voice to discover calmness and confidence. Toning can be seen as a type of armour that protects you throughout the day. Negative thoughts cling to the aura and can become tumours, cancers, etc. As you would take out the rubbish in your house, toning clears and restores the body. Keyes writes, 'Every word that we speak or sound that we make, sets in motion either harmony or discord in our lives'[1].

Exercises

1. When we are content, we naturally hum. Try humming more consciously and feel what happens inside your body. Try: 'MMMMM', 'NNNNN', 'OOOOO'. Then: 'moo-maa-maa'.

2. Then hum and/or sing an old song or poem. Or chant:

> *Seated at home behold me,*
> *Seated amid the rainbow,*
> *Seated at home.*
> *Lo, here in this holy place.*
> *Yes, seated at home, behold me.*
> *In life unending and beyond it,*
> *Yes seated at home, behold me!*
> *In joy unchanging,*
> *Yes, seated at home, behold me.*[2]

3. Close your eyes and inwardly watch your breath slow to about four times a minute. Say to yourself: 'Each time I take a breath I renew and restore my body and mind'. See your body filling up with light. If you feel any tension or darkness, let it out with a sigh or a groan. Visualise your higher self as a large halo above your head. See the halo moving down and touching your head. This is the symbol of enlightenment. What do you hear or see?

4. Try chanting this Sai Baba mantra[3]: Satya Dharma Shanti Prema (meaning Truth, The Path, Peace, Love). Repeat it five times.

Singing mantras is an ancient and well-documented method of liberating your awareness. They are very simple utterances. 'OM' is the most familiar. It acts as a link between the earthly and heavenly realms. One way to begin to access spirit is to listen to nature. Become aware of the sound of the birds, the grasshoppers, rushing water. . . If you live in an urban environment, you could purchase a tape of natural sounds which will remind you of the natural world. As you meditate on these sounds you begin to become aware of the body's inner sounds. Listen to your breath, the beating of your heart ...

Heart sound exercise

Try tuning into the sounds of your heart. Hum or sing a vowel sound such as 'ooo'. Slowly allow your voice to glide upward. Pause and breathe as you need to. Do not hurry. As the sound rises in pitch, imagine that it is also rising upwards from the base of your spinal column. At certain points along the musical slide you may be able to sense a reaction, maybe. pressure, heat or cold.

If singing or chanting interests you try and see if

you can attend a course with one of the people listed at the end of the chapter. Mantras and chanting systems are best when taught by a skilled teacher. It is difficult to realise the full potential of the energy transfer that goes with receiving a mantra when you are attempting to learn it on your own.

Music, particularly classical music, has a powerful healing ability. The prophet Nostradamus[4] predicted that there would be a cure for cancer found through sound therapy at this time. The break through has not yet happened, however, Steve Hellaby writes: 'There is current research on cancer cells which indicates that sounds around the note A above middle C (440 cycles per second) disrupt cancer cells but leave normal cells intact'[5]. Contact New Approaches to Cancer for more advice on this. Steve also has a chakra balancing tape, 'Chakra Tuning and Harmonic Meditation', to try.

[1] Elizabeth Laurel Keyes,*Toning: the creative power of the voice*, California: Marina del Rey, 1973, p. 40.

[2] Olivea Dewhurst-Maddock, *The Book of Sound Therapy: heal yourself with music and voice*, London: Gaia Books, 1993, p. 63.

[3] 'Mantra' is a Sanskrit word meaning 'the thought that liberates and protects'.

[4] Nostradamus, or Michel de Nostredame, was born in 1503 in Provence.

[5] Reference: Steve Hellaby, *Sound Therapy*, Egham: New Approaches to Cancer, 1993.

Books for further reading

Jonathan Goldman, *Healing Sounds: the power of harmonics*, Shaftesbury: Element, 1992.
(Goldman is director of The Sound Healers Association.)

Patricia Joudry, *Sound Therapy for the Walkman*, Canada: Steele and Steele, 1989.

Laurel Elizabeth Keyes, *Toning: the creative power of the voice*, California: Marina del Rey, 1973.

Olivea Dewhurst-Maddock, *The Book of Sound Therapy: heal yourself with music and voice*, London: Gaia Books, 1993.

Useful addresses

Steve Hellaby, New Approaches to Cancer, 5 Larksfield, Englefield Green, Egham, Surrey TW20 0RB.

Chris James, Sounds Wonderful, 24 Brunswick Road, South-end-on-sea, Essex SS1 2UH.

Muzz Murray, Inner Garden, 105 Gales Drive, Three Bridges, Crawley, Sussex RH10 1QD.

Jill Purce, Inner Sound & Voice Workshops, 20 Willow Road, Hampstead NW13 1TJ.

Tomatis Therapy, The Marsden Centre, 30 Oliver Lane, Marsden, Huddersfield HD7 6BZ. (Sound Therapy for the Walkman)

I USE

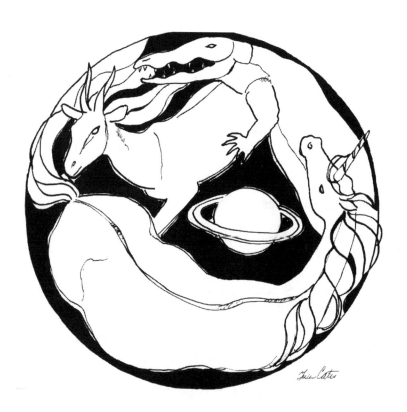

CAPRICORN
"Transition"

X

Spiritual healing

I looked up at the clouds, and two men were coming there, headfirst like arrows slanting down; and as they came, they sang a sacred song and the thunder was like drumming. I will sing it for you. The song and the drumming were like this:
> *'Behold a sacred voice is calling you;*
> *All over the sky a sacred voice is calling.'*
> *– Black Elk*

Throughout history, certain people have had the ability to cure disease and ease pain simply by placing their hands on the afflicted part of the body. Sometimes various remedies and incantations are also used. A healer has the ability to 'tune in' or establish a mental or physical rapport with the sick person. Spiritual healing is not a logical form of treatment and is, at times, in direct contradiction to medical science. However, when reviewing case studies, it becomes apparent that permanent results are often achieved by healers.

Clinical research shows that body and mind are indivisible. Now we are seeing that many disorders are due to emotional or mental factors. A spiritual healer takes this one step further, believing that the spiritual and physical are also interrelated.

A healer does not try to replace a medical doctor's role, but has a simpler goal: to restore balance and harmony where there is sickness and pain. Like other practitioners, the healer attempts to stimulate a natural and innate process of self-healing. A healer's equipment is the natural source of energy that surrounds her[1]. Healers administer treatments in different ways, but they normally agree that the source of natural energy from which their healing is derived is from God or some sort of Universal Energy. They also tend to agree that unconditional love is an important factor in their work.

Many spiritual healers work with hands on contact, but others work just as effectively at a distance. Through prayer and meditation, the healer initiates a healing process. Sometimes the results are instantaneous, but usually healing is a gradual process.

Some of the more common phenomena associated with spiritual healing is the slow dispersal of tumours and cancerous growths. There are many recorded accounts of spinal curvatures, particularly due to arthritis, straightening under the healer's hands. Osteo-adhesions, prolapsed discs and duodenal (intestinal) ulcers often respond well to spiritual healing.

A 'divine healer' is often orthodox in her beliefs. This gives a wholly religious approach to healing. It involves the forgiveness of sin, implying that the patient's sickness is the direct result of her failure to realise the Christian ideals of living. This can cause great psychological damage. Luckily, in recent years the church has become more realistic in its ministry of healing. We are beginning to realise that the religious aspects of healing only reveal a limited understanding of the nature of the forces involved. Part of the New Age awareness is about helping us see that regardless of age, race, class, sex or religion, we all are one.

A healer offers both patient and medical practitioner a different view of the causes and cures of disease. The process also tends to awaken the patient's innate self-healing abilities. To the healer, health is not restricted to the physical body, but also takes into consideration our mental and emotional states. The healing process involves remembering who you truly are. It may involve experiencing regression or far memory, a technique that helps the patients remember their past lives. This type of inner healing helps the patients focus on their belief systems and the reality they have created for themselves. It also empowers them to change their reality. A healer may also work with the different layers of the aura[2], including the physical body systems, through the laying on of hands.

An example of spiritual healing

Betty experienced psychological abuse in childhood. However, she has reached a stage in her life when she is ready to let those feelings go so that they no longer effect her life. The healer uses counselling skills to help Betty see the experience from an adult perspective. On the emotional level, the healer helps Betty clear blocked feelings. The healer works on the aura to re-establish a sense of well-being and strength. The healer then intuitively (using a pendulum) suggests a diet, food supplements (vitamins and minerals) and yoga to help Betty continue this process on her own.

Some people are born with a natural gift for healing. It tends to be a feminine trait; however, the gift is within us all. There tends to be a battle within most of us between the ego and the spirit. This is a necessary battle since we are here to learn about earthly existence. Spirit is free. It knows no boundaries and has no fear. It is not physical. Spirit thinks it can do anything. Ego, on the other hand, is the critical voice that we hear that reminds us of our limitations. When we get ready to walk down a dark alley at night, ego says that it might not be a good idea. Ego saves us. However, if we listen only to ego our world becomes very limited and very frightening. Ego does not like the idea of poverty, disease or death. None of this frightens spirit because it knows it is immortal. Ego is linked to the intellect and has become the favoured type of thought. What we really need is a balance between the two.

Spirit, or our intuitive voice, is our creativity. Children are in touch with this energy. You know spirit is present when you feel light, when you laugh for no reason, when you are in a state of bliss. Others can try to convince you of a whole assortment of things, but if you are laughing, then you are on your way to becoming whole. A good way to begin to distinguish between these two types of thought is to recognise them while writing.

Ego–spirit exercise

Take out two pieces of paper. Write 'ego' on the top of one sheet with a brown crayon or pen. Write 'spirit' on the top of the other with a blue crayon or pen. Use a third piece of paper to begin on. Take a deep breath. Imagine your body filling with white light. When you feel ready, begin to write anything that comes into your head. At first there will probably just be some superficial stuff coming out about how you are feeling and how much your brother irritates you, or whatever. Keep going. Don't think. What you will eventually hit is an interesting stream of information. This is the subconscious, the realm of dreams. This is spirit, so write it on the 'spirit' sheet. Every time a negative thought comes into your head such as: 'I'm such an idiot, I can't spell and my teacher at school said . . .', write it on the 'ego' sheet. That is your limitation. What this exercise can do is help you break through this type of restriction and get back in touch with your true self that has all the knowledge you need. When you hear words that encourage and support, know that they come from the world of spirit. Let go – what does spirit have to say?

Healing exercise

This exercise helps you tap into your innate healing ability. Practice first with a plant, then, when you are comfortable, with a pet and then on a friend.

Close your eyes and take a deep breath. See your body filling up with white light. Visualise a cord running from your feet deep into the earth. See the dark richness of the earth, the rocks and hidden streams. Eventually you reach the middle of the earth where you find a large glowing crystal. Attach the cord to the crystal and feel the wonderful healing energies that emanate from it. Then travel quickly back to your body taking the earth's healing power with you. Pull this red energy up to your navel. Then visualise a cord coming out the back of your neck just beneath your skull and follow it skyward into a spiral tunnel. Travel quickly to the sun. Feel his golden healing energies. Then travel back down the tunnel taking some healing rays with you. Know that your body is filled with healing energies.

Place your hands towards a plant so that your fingertips point upwards and your palms face the plant. See yourself pulling the healing energy from the earth up into your shoulders and out your hands so that rainbows of light are offered from the earth to the plant. See the healing light from the sun (or God) running through your head and neck and out your hands as a beautiful white light. See the earth and sun energies merging and dancing together. Visualise this energy being sent directly to the plant. When you feel the plant has had all it needs, close your eyes and ask that this light be shared with whoever needs it this day. Know that the light flows through you, but does not come from you. You are merely a helper in the process and your intent is to channel light for the good of all. Know that whatever healing needs to take place will take place, and that is all.

Gently release the cords from your feet and neck. Know you can pull them towards you any time you wish. Then visualise a blue cloak that you place over your body to protect yourself from outside influences. Know you are safe.

It is necessary to wash your hands with cold water between healings and afterwards. It washes away any negativity you may have collected from the recipient and reminds you to completely detach from their energy field. You have acted as a channel for the light; the way they choose to utilise that energy is their decision.

---

[1] Since most healers are women, I have used the feminine form for the sake of clarity. Please remember the gender is interchangeable.
[2] See Section IV on Energy therapies.

Books for further reading

Barbara Brennan, *Hands of Light: a guide to healing through the human energy field*, London: Bantam, 1987.

LaUna Huffines, *Bridge of Light: tools of light for spiritual transformation*, California: Kramer, 1993.

Stanley Krippner and Villoldo, *The Realms of Healing*, California: Celestial Arts, 1976.

Rudolf Steiner, *Colour*, Bristol: Rudolph Steiner Press, 1992.

Useful addresses:

The National Federation of Spiritual Healers, Old Manor Farm Studio, Church Street, Kingston-on-Thames, Middlesex TW16 6RG.

I KNOW

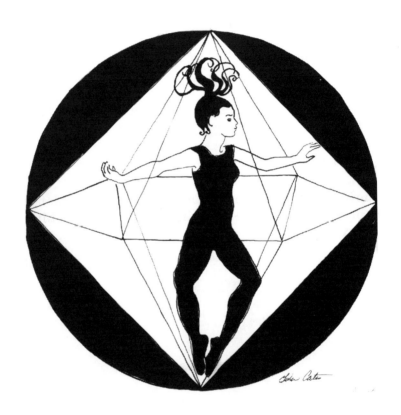

AQUARIUS
"Crystal Pirouette"

XI

Visualisation: the power of positive thought

*Meditation leads us to the inner work place.
Meditation is a creative act that can lead us to
the place where the pilot light of the flame of life
burns at all times...*
– Jack Schwarz

Many people within the field of alternative psychology
recognise that our mental attitude plays a large role in
determining our experiences. Basically, what you think
will happen, will happen. We create our own realities.
That is why it is so important to do daily affirmations. The
word 'affirm' comes from the Latin affirmare meaning 'to
make firm'. When we visualise we are using our minds
to consciously create what we want. If you want to be
healthy, tell yourself you are healthy. Do not say you want
to be healthy, because that implies that your health will
be found in the future, therefore it may not happen. The
affirmation must take place in the present. If you need to
make money, affirm that you are wealthy and that money
comes easily to you. What ever it is that you want tell
yourself that it is happening now. Write it down on a piece
of paper and remind yourself of it again and again until
you are totally convinced it is a reality. Love yourself;
know you can do it. Remember, love is the most powerful force on earth.

Meditation

Meditation is a form of mental exercise designed to
expand your awareness. However, like physical exercise,
commitment is required if one expects to achieve results.
Meditation is a discipline that teaches us to relax the body

and quiet the mind so that we may find the divine spark within. Once you have become disciplined in the art of meditation, interesting things begin to happen in your life. When you are meditating you turn within. In that world, action and desire cease to exist. What then happens is that instead of pushing what you want away from you, what you want is allowed to happen. The external world of circumstances and possibilities stops expanding. Because of your introspection, circumstances and possibilities come back towards you. Therefore your hopes and dreams come in closer and closer until they become an actual physical reality. This can only happen when you become emotionally detached and allow things to happen. It takes a great deal of discipline. But this is what people mean when they say, 'let go and let God'. It's basically getting off your case so you can allow the goodness and abundance into your life that is your natural inheritance.

There are several disciplines involved when we begin. First we must set aside time each day for meditation, preferably at a fixed hour. Second we must learn to sit still and relax the body. Third we must quiet the mind. This requires silencing the internal dialogues that usually occupy our minds. When we meditate, we learn to master our mind. If we do not control the mind, it is unlikely that we will realise our own true self. There are many ways of practising mind control, they include: (1) passive meditation (for example, concentration on the breath) and (2) active meditation when we take advantage of the conscious energy of the mind through the controlled use of our imaginations (for instance, visualisation).

Visualisation: the power of positive thought

Find a quiet and warm place where you will not be disturbed. Light a candle and dedicate it to the path or deity you follow (for instance, 'God' or 'the beings of goodness and light'). Sit on a chair or in a comfortable position on the floor with your back against the wall. Make sure your spine is straight. Let go of any thoughts that enter your mind, let them drift away like soap bubbles.

When stress becomes a part of our lives, it creates pressure on both the brain and body, which in turn creates physical and mental problems that can be difficult to heal. The following meditation allows the negative congestion that can build up in the body to be dispersed. Try the following exercise after telling yourself that there is always a safety key (I use the image of a little magical cloud) at your command any time you want to opt out. You could record this onto a cassette tape and then play it to yourself:

Meditation: the cloud

1. Sit or lie down. Make yourself comfortable but try not to fall asleep. Imagine yourself in a sunlit garden. Feel the warmth of the sun pervading every part of your body, from your toes to the top of your head.

2. Walk down to the end of the garden. There is a great oak tree. You climb easily and lightly up into its branches and up to the top of the tree.

3. Here you find a little cloud waiting for you. Does your friend the cloud have a name? Climb into the soft, fluffy cloud and allow yourself to travel through the sky. You can control the speed yourself. Remember, the cloud will take you straight home any time you want to quit.

4. The cloud brings you gently back to earth and you find yourself slipping into a warm swimming pool filled with salty water. You feel yourself floating on the surface. Do not try to swim.

5. (When you are in this relaxed state, auto-suggestion is very powerful. Tell yourself that you do not wish to smoke, overeat, worry, etc. In this state you can convince your subconscious of anything! However, make sure your intention is correct. Always suggest things to yourself that will bring you into a state of harmony and balance.) Say aloud, 'I am healthy. I am happy. I am wealthy. I am free!' or anything else you feel you need to tell yourself at this time.

6. When you feel that you have spent enough time in your pool, simply ask your cloud to take you home. Climb aboard and it will carry you back to the top of the tree. You climb back down the branches to earth with ease.

7. Walk back to the garden and lie down on the spot where you started your journey. Perhaps you would like to mark it with a flower.

Remember your mental safety key (the cloud) and that you can choose to stop the exercise at any time. It may take a little while before you feel comfortable doing the whole exercise, but perseverance will pay off. Once the exercise has been completed, you will have a mental key that you can use any time.

When walking in the countryside or planting herbs in your garden, it is good to acknowledge and thank the elementals who are responsible for the elements of earth (the gnomes), water (the undines), fire (the salamanders) and air (the sylphs). If we ask for their help and thank them for helping us, they will become our friends and servants. If we misuse them, they can create havoc.

Find a quiet and comfortable place to sit where you will not be disturbed. Remember to take the telephone off the hook. If possible, sit on a pillow on the floor with your legs out straight or cross-legged with your back supported. This is a special time for you. Light a candle and dedicate it to the path you are now following. Keep your spine straight:

Meditation: thanking the elementals

See your spine as a golden shaft of light that earths you to this planet and also lifts you up to higher dimensions. Let go of any thoughts that come into your mind. Remember to protect yourself with white light before and after meditation.

Imagine that you are standing at the end of a narrow and dimly lit corridor. Slowly you start to walk down this corridor. You feel the unevenness of the floor beneath your feet and you notice that the walls are made of rock which is rough and jagged to touch. The further down the corridor you walk, the dimmer the light becomes. There is just enough light for you to see the door that you are approaching. It is made of oak and has a round wooden handle on its right-hand side. You take hold of the handle, sensing the smoothness and warmth of the wood and turn it, opening the door outwards.

As you walk through the doorway, you find yourself in the countryside. It is still dark and everything is still and silent. Lifting your gaze upwards, you look into a star-filled sky which twinkles and shines like hundreds of precious jewels. Above, there is a bright crescent moon which is surrounded by luminous colours.

You find a path in front of you and you start to walk along it. You feel the stones and gravel beneath your feet. Some feel smooth, others sharp. You remember with gratitude the elementals who are responsible for the mineral kingdom, the gnomes. In remembering these elementals, your thoughts turn to the beautiful crystals which are formed in the darkness of the earth, the white of the diamond through to the red of the ruby. You are reminded that out of the sacred darkness comes light.

Step off the gravel path and onto the grass. The grass has a different texture, it feels smooth and soft, with a slightly colder sensation. You become aware that different parts of your feet pick up different sensations. Stop for a moment and look at the surrounding trees. Although they are still cloaked in darkness, you can still feel their majesty. They seem to be inviting you to share the energy that they absorbed during the day. As you stand and look with awe and wonder, the sound of distant water reaches you. Its rippling, bubbling music invites you to walk towards it. The sound grows louder as you approach the river whose water dances its way across the countryside. On its banks is a tethered boat. Get into it and allow the river to carry you along. Lying back in the boat, you sense that dawn is just about to break. Behind you, the sky is still a deep indigo, but as you move your gaze towards the horizon, the indigo turns to a pale blue. Placing your hand over the side of the boat and into the water, you feel a tingling coldness. The water seems to wash away any tension in your hand, leaving it relaxed and refreshed. Gliding gently along, you remember with thankfulness the elementals who are responsible for the element of water, the undines.

Slowly your boat drifts into a small bay and stops. You get out and secure it to a mooring post. See the sun rising over the horizon. Dawn has almost broken. In front of you stands a magnolia tree laden with magenta blossoms. Sit beneath its boughs and absorb its colours into your being. Breathe in its delicate perfume. A gentle breeze softly rustles its green leaves and plays around your hair and face. Yellow rays of light shine forth from behind the tree, reminding you of the elementals of air, the sylphs, and you thank them.

Dawn has now fully broken and the sun glows a golden orange on the horizon. Farm animals and birds have awakened to this new day and sing and call to each other. The noise of farm-hands starting their work travels across the countryside. You feel the warmth from the newly risen sun radiating on your body and energising every cell and atom. In thankfulness you remember the salamanders, the elementals who are responsible for the element of fire. Your whole being starts to radiate peace, tranquillity and love. Stop to take in the red essence of a red rose in full blossom. Feel that you are part of the earth.

Realising that it is time to return home, slowly stand up and look around you. You notice that the boat in which you have travelled has brought you in almost a complete circle and that just a few yards in front of where you are sitting is the door through which you came.

Stand up and walk to the door, turn the handle and open the door towards you. Walk through it, back into the corridor. After the brilliance of the dawn, the corridor seems very dark and narrow. Continue to walk along the corridor until you enter the room where you started this meditation. Become aware of your body. In your mind's eye, lie down on the spot where you started your journey. Stretch your toes, then your hands, legs and arms. Feel yourself back in your body. Please look down before looking up.[1]

Lunar cycles and full moon meditation

> *So make a lantern,*
> *Lit from the Red Indian fire*
> *And whose light shines clear*
> *For the way you've come*
> *To be seen and marked,*
> *And the way ahead to hold no fear*
> *For others who come after you*
> *To walk with an assurance,*
> *Seeing by light from a torch you have left ...*

> *– from The Commission Given to Flying Horse*
> *by the Mystic Medicine Chief Silver Bear*

During its orbit of approximately twenty-nine days round the earth, the moon has a tremendous effect on all living creatures. Moon cycles have a powerful influence on water. More than 70% of the earth's surface is water. Water is present in everything on earth, since there is no life without it. The moon's magnetic force causes the rise and fall of the ocean's tides. It influences the flow of sap in trees and plants. This gravitational pull effects all things, including the human body, since we too are composed of 70% water. The moon effects the rhythm of blood, female menstruation and gestation. Moon cycles even effect the fluids in the brain.

To the Native American all of life seemed to operate in circular patterns. They regarded the medicine wheel as the symbol of the universe. Man looked out through the eye which was round and saw the circular planets that surrounded the earth. The rising and setting of the sun followed a circular pattern, as did the seasons. Birds built their homes in circular nests and animals marked their territories in circles. In the old days, Indian tribes lived in tepees with a circular base. To the Indian the circle was the principal symbol for understanding life's mysteries.

As we become more aware of our own cycles, we begin to find our connection with the cycles of nature. There are four stages of the moon. The first stage is the dark moon. At this time the moon is not visible because it is rising in the same place as the sun. This four day phase is followed by the thin crescent of the new moon. The dark moon is a time of rest; a time for contemplation, but not action. The new moon, as the tide of energies begins to increase, is the time to begin new projects.

The second phase is called the waxing moon. At this time the size of the moon increases over an eleven day period. Energies are flowing fast and it is a time to plant things that grow towards the light. It is also the time to work on attracting things into our lives.

The third stage is the full moon which lasts three days. At this time the moon is a completed circle and her light is at its brightest. It is a time for completing projects. There is an increase in the energy and activity within nature. It is a good time to meditate.

The fourth stage is the waning moon. At this time the moon begins to diminish in size. After eleven days it is reduced to a narrow crescent and the cycle begins again. During the waning moon energies are flowing away like the ebb of the sea tide. It is a time of giving to others and of planting crops that grow downwards.

Full moon meditation

During the time of the full moon, groups of people around the world work together in meditation asking that light stream forth into the world. Do this meditation close to the time of the full moon. Light a candle as a symbol of the light energies you now invite to enlighten earth.

If the moon is currently in a different phase, honour this time and see yourself as part of the cycle. Try to discover how you are working or can work with the phases of the moon. Go outside at night and look at the silvery reflection of the moon. Write your feelings and impressions at this time. Come back to this meditation when the moon is full.

This meditation should be read aloud, preferably with friends sharing the reading. If you have trouble with the word 'God', please feel free to change it to 'Allah', 'beings of goodness and light', or whatever deity you follow.

1. Realise that we are an energy centre, a centre of light. In a spirit of dedication we link with all other groups and individuals who are making their approach at this time of the full moon.

2. As we link on the mental plane, we visualise a network of light spreading all over the world bringing love to all living things.

3. We raise our consciousness to the Soul, the Christ within, which links us with the Heart of God and with the centre where the Will of God is known.

4. Holding our minds steady in the light, we visualise a stream of love pouring through into the hearts of men and women.

In the centre of all Love I stand;
From that centre I, the one who serves, will work.
May the love of the divine Self be shed abroad
In my heart, through my group, and throughout the world.

5. Let the soul control the outer form and life and all events. Let love prevail; let all men love.

SILENCE – 10 MINUTE MEDITATION

6. We transmit the tide of Love outward into the world of men and women, visualising the radiation of love creating lines of lighted relationships between all men and women, races and nations.

7. We will say THE GREAT INVOCATION[2] together:

From the point of Light within the Mind of God
Let Light stream forth into the minds of men.
Let Light descend on Earth.

From the point of Love within the Heart of God
Let love stream forth into the hearts of men.
May Christ return to Earth.

From the centre where the Will of God is known
Let purpose guide the little wills of men –
The purpose which the Masters know and serve.

From the centre which we call the race of men
Let the Plan of Love and Light work out
And may it seal the door where evil dwells.

Let Light and Love and Power restore the Plan on Earth.

---

[1] Based on a meditation by Pauline Wills.
[2] This information comes from the Lucis Trust. See useful addresses. Contact them if you would like to join or start your own full moon meditation group.

Books for further reading

Louise Hay, *You Can Heal Your Life*, London: Eden Grove Editions, 1988.

Louise Hay, *The Power Is Within You*, London: Eden Grove Editions, 1991.

Chris Odle, *Practical Visualization*, London: The Aquarian Press, 1990.

Stuart Wilde, *Whispering Winds of Change: perceptions of a new world*, Australia: Nacson & Sons, 1993.

Useful addresses

Lucis Trust, (Incorporating Arcane School, Triangles, World Goodwill) Suite 54, 3 Whitehall Court, London SW1A 2EF.

I BELIEVE

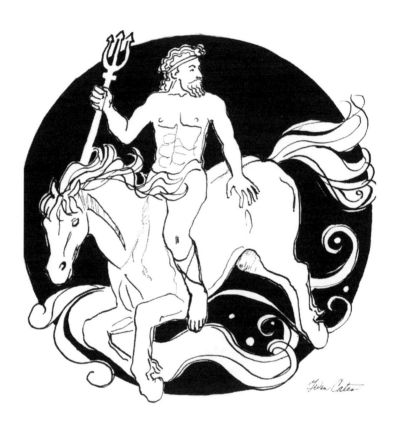

PISCES
"Riding the Waves"

XII

Yoga

When, as earth, water, light, heat, and ether arise, the fivefold quality of Yoga takes place, then there is no longer illness, old age, or pain for him who has obtained a body, produced by the fire of Yoga.
– Svetasvatara Upanishad

Yogis learn to listen to the body, observe its needs and adopt a friendly attitude toward it. This often results in recovering the alertness and swiftness that normally belongs to children. By doing yoga we learn to appreciate our body. We must all die eventually, however, none of us want the body to degenerate while we are alive. By doing yoga we are more likely to retain a state of suppleness and health until the end.

If an immune system problem such as cancer or AIDS has already developed within your body, yoga can be a useful tool to use in addition to your medical treatment. The British Medical Association has accepted that yoga is a complementary process[1]. That is, the BMA recognises the self-help benefits of yoga. As with all therapies, it is a good idea to consult an experienced practitioner. Although yoga in itself cannot cure cancer or other immune system disorders, it can help you face the many physical and emotional trials that illness brings. Yoga Nidra, a type of visualisation, can help you fight illness. Dr Bernie Siegel, the American cancer surgeon, is one of many who emphasises the importance of yoga.

Each yoga posture — *asana* — has specific benefits. Sometimes this is as simple as maintaining the suppleness of muscles and joints, encouraging increased circulation in the body and the massage of internal organs.

People who are very strict with their yogasanas, or body postures, often find that very soon their stamina and strength are increased. It is said that yoga performed correctly will lead to the complete control of all bodily functions. Researchers have found that yoga is especially beneficial for the following conditions: stress, depression, ME (myalgic encephalomyelitis), RSI (repetitive strain injury), low back pain, chest conditions (particularly blocked airways), arthritis, heart conditions[2] and neuro-muscular conditions such as multiple sclerosis and Parkinson's disease.[3]

The different types of yoga

The word 'yoga' is derived from the root word 'yug' or 'yuj' meaning 'to join' or 'to unite'. Behind the discipline of yoga is the wish to unite body, mind and spirit. Yoga is not associated with any particular religious or metaphysical establishment[4]. The two most widely practised forms of yoga in the West are Hatha Yoga and Raja Yoga. Hatha Yoga is also known as the 'yoga of vitality' or physiological yoga. Hatha Yoga is characterised by the disciplines of various postures and breath control. Raja or Royal Yoga is the yoga of mental mastery, or the 'yoga of meditation'. It is aimed at union with the One (or God).

Hatha Yoga, the most practical of yogas, is designed to strengthen the physical body, fight against disease and ward off death. It also has a grounding and calming influence on the mind. All Hatha Yoga exercises involve regulation of the breath and harmonisation of sun (male energies) and moon (female energies). The flow from the right nostril is known as 'sun breath' and the flow from the left nostril is known as 'moon breath'. The control and regulation of breath helps to balance the whole being.

Asana originally meant 'sitting method' or 'seat'.

This type of yoga is practised in the West generally because of its great health benefits. Asanas are known to strengthen the nervous system, glands and vital organs.

Raja Yoga is closely associated with Patanjali and his *Yoga Sutras*. Raja Yoga is seen as a type of physiological hygiene, preparing the body for effective mental control. It works upon the mind, refining and perfecting it. Through the mind, it heals the body.

Yoga is an ancient technique that has been tried and tested over many thousands of years. Again and again people have found that through tuning the body and the mind one is able to bring health to the body, calmness to the mind and find balance and harmony in daily existence; some followers even find a deeper peace after glimpsing the light (samadhi or intuitive enlightenment). Yoga is a wonderful way to reduce the stress imposed upon us by the modern world. People of all ages, races and genders can practice yoga. Our bodies have different needs. Remember to allow your body to be your guide.

The corpse posture

All yoga techniques are designed to produce tranquillity. This relaxing influence is probably yoga's greatest gift to Western man. Simply playing dead in the corpse posture (savasana) has great restorative powers. It effectively eases fatigue and quiets the mind. Try this 'letting go' exercise:

Lie flat on your back, with your legs outstretched and your heels a little way apart. Allow your feet to fall limply outwards. Your arms should lie along your body, resting on the floor with the palm of your hands turned upwards. Allow the fingers to be limp and slightly curled. If you feel uncomfortable, place cushions below your neck and/or each knee.

Turn your attention to your breath. Make sure you are breathing out of your nostrils, not your mouth. Do not alter your breath, simply observe it. Then take a deep abdominal breath, exhale fully. Repeat. See the abdomen swelling out like a balloon on the inhalation, and then on the exhalation visualise yourself pushing the abdominal muscles back toward the spine. Then release the abdominal muscles, and once again turn your attention to the rise and fall of your normal respiration. You will find that your breathing becomes smooth and regular. Occasionally you may want to take in a deep breath and let out a sigh. That is fine. It is simply a sign that tension is being released somewhere in your body.

Now that you feel calm and your breathing is relaxed, focus your attention like a torch beam and read your body from feet to head, looking for tension. If you find any tension, let out a sigh and feel it leaving you. Feel what happens when the mind silently commands 'let go'. Immediately the tension is released. When you can no longer feel any more tension in your body, enjoy the sensation. Do you feel like a baby, or perhaps a cat? Enjoy the freedom of total relaxation. Remember how quickly the body obeyed suggestion. Do you see how you create your own ease or dis-ease? You are the creator of your reality. Enjoy it.

When you are ready, roll onto your side and become aware of your body again. Wiggle your toes and then your fingers. Stretch up the left side of your body and then the right. Stretch your whole body. Slowly sit up.

More yoga

The forest sages of old sat immobile for hours. Out of this developed a series of postures to be held for a few seconds, minutes or hours. The asanas are designed to discipline the body and mind in order to master the body's health. Some postures copy the birds, animals, reptiles and insects after which they were named.

In 1896–7 a yogi presented a series of postures in London and was considered a freak. However, by the 1950s there was a growing tolerance and acceptance of yoga. Today, since research has shown it brings worthwhile results, yoga is very popular. Asanas are designed to be refreshing. Yoga is non-competitive and requires no special equipment. It can be performed by men, women and children of all ages.

Yoga is best done three hours after a main meal or one hour after a light snack. Remember to empty your bladder and bowels before exercising. Wear loose-fitting clothing made of natural fibres. Perform your postures on a firm floor on a blanket, rug or mat (the non-slip kind is best). If you are in generally good health try the following exercises. Otherwise see what you feel comfortable doing.

British Wheel of Yoga 1st Sequence[5]

1. Stand up. Feel as though a string is attached to the top of your head and is pulling you up so that you stand perfectly straight. Make sure that your weight is evenly balanced over both feet and that your feet are pelvic-width apart. Allow your arms to rest by your sides.

2. Slowly raise your arms out to the side and then above your head, pause, and lower them. Repeat. This time breathe in as you raise your arms and breathe out as you lower them. (Allow a little more weight to rest in your heels as you perform this exercise.)

3. The *Rag Doll Stand*: Stand tall, then slowly begin to sway from side to side. Feel yourself freeing up all the joints in your body from your feet to the top of your head. When you feel free and loose, turn and look round to the left,

then round to the right, allowing the arms to swing. Go slowly to begin with and, if there is no dizziness, quicken if you wish.

4. Stand with your feet apart, raising first the right arm and stretching the right side of the body from the outside of the right foot to the right finger tips. Repeat on the other side. To extend the movement, breathe in as you raise your arm, breathe out as you lower it.

5. *Forward bend*: Stand tall. Bend the knees a little then fold forward from the hip joints to keep the spine long. Then roll up, one vertebrae at a time, into standing position.

6. *The Tree*: This posture is designed to help your balance. (If your balance is not good, stand close to a wall.) Find something solid on the wall in front of you, like a picture frame or beam, to look at. Focusing on it will help you find your balance. Stand tall with your weight on your right foot. Put the sole of your left foot to the inside of the right ankle, your big toe touching the floor and your left knee out to the side. Then put your hands together into a prayer position. Breathe easily and hold the posture for five to ten breaths. Repeat on the other side. If your balance is good, you can try taking the foot further up the inside of the leg.

7. *The Squat*: Stand tall with your feet together. Come up on your toes and bring your hands to shoulder level. Then bend slowly till you are sitting on your heels with your hands by your sides. Return slowly to standing. Repeat. If you feel comfortable, extend this posture by breathing in as you raise your arms and going up on your toes and breathing out as you squat down.

8. *The Cat*: Come forward on to your hands and knees. Make sure your knees are hip-width apart and that your arms are in alignment with your shoulders. To do the pos-

ture, lower your abdomen towards the floor and look forward. Pause. Then raise the spine towards the ceiling as you lower your head between your arms. You will look like a cat stretching its back. Repeat the exercise, but this time try adding breath control. Breathe in as you lower the abdomen and look forward. Then breathe out as you raise your spine and lower your head. Repeat.

9. *The Cobra*: Lie face downward on the floor with legs a little apart and pelvis comfortable. Place your hands shoulder-width apart a little beyond the head. Put your forehead on the floor. Using the lower back muscles first, start to raise the upper part of your body from the floor, then use your hands to continue the stretch. Hold the position while looking forward. Count to three, then return slowly to the floor. Repeat.

10. *Spinal Rock*: Sit on the floor with knees bent. Bend your chin towards your chest. Wrap your arms around your legs and rock gently backwards on to your back. Hold your legs firmly and rock back and forth. Rest, then repeat.

11. *Half Shoulder stand*: Begin as you would for the spinal rock. Rock well back and as the buttocks come off the floor, put your hands under your lower back and support your body. Straighten your legs towards the ceiling. Hold the position for five to ten breaths, if possible, before rocking back to sitting.

12. *Breathing Meditation*: Find a comfortable sitting position. Relax. Allow your breathing to settle into a natural rhythm. Turn your full attention to the rise and fall of your breath. Do not alter the breath, just be aware of it. Count each inspiration from one to ten, then go back to one. This focuses the attention and does not allow the mind to wander. If thoughts come into your mind let them go. Repeat.

13. *The Corpse*: (As described earlier.) It is a good idea to

put on some extra clothing or have a blanket to cover yourself. From sitting position uncurl your body onto the floor. Slowly straighten your legs, spreading them slightly apart. Place your arms by your sides, palms facing upwards. Lift your head, look down your body to see if it is in line. Then rest your head. Feel that the back of your neck is stretched and the chin is pointing towards the chest. Remember it is important to feel comfortable, so use some cushions if necessary.

14 . *Heartbeat Meditation*: Keep your eyes closed. Relax. Listen to your heartbeat. Focus on its rhythm. It is the pulse of life. (Pause.) Continue to count for five to ten minutes. Then roll on to your side. Rest for a moment.

---

[1] Reference: Yoga for Health Foundation.

[2] A programme headed by Dr Dean Ornish, involving regular yoga, diet, exercise and mental co-ordination, has been shown in controlled trials to reverse heart disease.

[3] For more information contact Yoga for Health Foundation. This Foundation is a residential course centre founded in 1978 for the study and practice of therapeutic yoga. Over 20,000 people have stayed there. The centre provides training programmes and is also equipped to accommodate those with physical disability.

[4] The exception to the rule is Bhakti Yoga which is often presented with various types of Hindu mysticism.

[5] Reference: Pat Chittananda (Swami Sat Chidananda), *An Introduction to Yoga*, Lincs: British Wheel of Yoga, pp. 4–6.

Books for further reading

Alain, *Yoga For Perfect Health*, London: Thorsons, 1957.

James Hewitt, *The Complete Book of Yoga: yoga of breathing, yoga of posture, yoga of meditation*, London: Cresset Press, 1990.

Dr R. Nagarathna, Dr H.R. Nagendra and Dr Robin Monro, *Yoga for Common Ailments*, London: Gaia Books, 1990.

Vanda Scaravelli, *Awakening the Spine: the stress-free new yoga that restores health, vitality and energy*, London: Aquarian, 1991.

Magazines and pamphlets for further reading

'The Therapeutic Value of Yoga', Bedfordshire: Yoga For Health Foundation.

Pat Chittananda (Swami Sat Chidananda), 'An Introduction to Yoga', Lincs: British Wheel of Yoga.

'Yoga and Health' is a monthly publication covering a broad range of topics. Write: 21 Caburn Crescent, Lewes, East Sussex BN7 1NR.

Useful addresses

British Wheel of Yoga, 1 Hamilton Place, Boston Road, Sleaford, Lincolnshire NG34 7ES.

Yoga Biomedical Trust, 156 Cockerell Road, Cambridge CB4 3RZ.

Yoga for Health Foundation, Ickwell Bury, Biggleswade, Bedfordshire SG18 9EF. Tel: 01767-627271.

Consider this —

You believe divine oneness sees and judges people. We think of divine oneness as feeling the intent and the emotion of beings. Not as interested in what we do as why we do it.
–Marlo Morgan

You can create the reality that you want. We are here to experiment; everything we choose to do is fine as long as it doesn't hurt anyone else. If you do cause injury, sit quietly and think about it. When you feel you understand the reason, accept the situation, send the person love and let it go. Acting in a loving way doesn't mean that we let other people impose limitations on us. It means that we walk in the feeling of LOVE. Unconditional love, that is love without judgement or criticism, is very empowering. Unconditional love is the key to our freedom. Love has many descriptions, but it is a word you must feel to understand.

Do this meditation and *feel* what happens

Imagine that you are surrounded by a sphere of white light. See that white light penetrating you until you are one with the light. Then take an imaginary crayon and draw around the etheric field (the etheric field surrounds the entire body by about a quarter inch) as though you were drawing a silhouette. See yourself stand up. Visualise yourself standing in front of you. Then dance, or throw a fit, or find yourself performing whatever emotional activity you feel drawn into. Then find a feeling of peace once more. Let it all go ... Visualise a tunnel leading up into the sky. Find yourself being drawn into it. You are travelling so quickly you may feel dizzy. Marvel at the incredible speed at which you can travel. Then suddenly you come to the end of the tunnel. What you see before you is a huge ball of bright light, perhaps the only thing you will be able to compare it to is the sun. Realise that is your true self. Walk into the white light and realise you are home. Feel the warmth and joy that fills your entire being. Imagine that you have an ice cream scoop and that you have been allowed to take pieces of this wonderful bright light and direct it towards certain individuals. See hundreds of tunnels leading from the light to certain individuals that you know need this light. Imagine yourself tossing it into the tunnels and see it entering their hearts. Visualise their hearts lighting up like bright stars. Then see all the people that disturb you; people you have quarrelled with, or that you have unresolved issues with. (Remember we are karmically linked to all those we both love and hate. In order to release these ties that bind us, we must learn to forgive and let go.) See yourself sending light to all those people as well and see difficult situations being dissolved by the power of LOVE. Send light to any other people or places that may need it at this time. Then see the earth surrounded by this wonderful light. Realise that this light is eternal and that no matter how much you give away it never diminishes in size. See yourself radiating like the sun and realise that any time you need to visit you may. Now see yourself leaving and re-entering the tube. You quickly slide back into your body. Take your crayon and re-trace the etheric field around your body and realise that you have come back. Feel your breath. Listen to the wind, to the birds, to any small sounds you may hear. Remember how wonderful it is to be alive and to be experimenting in the physical plane. When you are ready open your eyes.

Index